NIKSEN

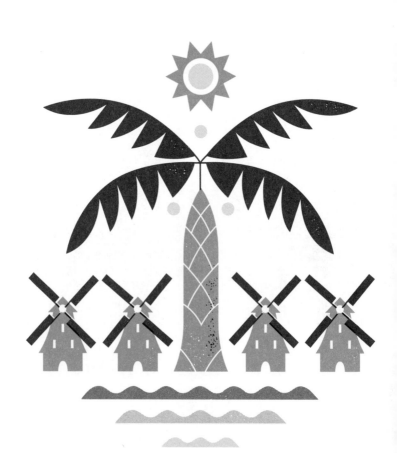

NIKSEN

Embracing the Dutch Art of Doing Nothing

OLGA MECKING

Houghton Mifflin Harcourt
Boston   New York
2021

For information about permission to reproduce selections
from this book, write to trade.permissions@hmhco.com or to
Permissions, Houghton Mifflin Harcourt Publishing Company,
3 Park Avenue, 19th Floor, New York, New York 10016.

hmhbooks.com

Library of Congress Cataloging-in-Publication Data
Names: Mecking, Olga, author.
Title: Niksen : embracing the Dutch art of doing nothing /
Olga Mecking.
Description: Boston : Houghton Mifflin Harcourt, 2021. |
Includes bibliographical references and index.
Identifiers: LCCN 2020033835 (print) | LCCN 2020033836 (ebook) |
ISBN 9780358395317 (hardback) | ISBN 9780358396352 |
ISBN 9780358396376 | ISBN 9780358395089 (ebook)
Subjects: LCSH: Conduct of life. | Well-being. | Relaxation. |
Stress (Physiology) | National characteristics, Dutch. |
Nothing (Philosophy) — Miscellanea.
Classification: LCC BJ1589 .M46 2021 (print) |
LCC BJ1589 (ebook) | DDC 155.8/9492 — dc23
LC record available at https://lccn.loc.gov/2020033835
LC ebook record available at https://lccn.loc.gov/2020033836

Book design by Chrissy Kurpeski

Printed in the United States of America
DOC 10 9 8 7 6 5 4 3 2 1

Contents

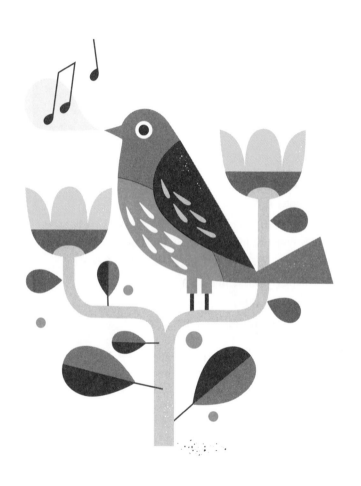

Oh No, Not Another Wellness Trend!

I'm on my couch, pondering a typical day in my life. Each morning I am awakened — right on time — by the sound of joyfully chirping birds. Before I get out of bed, I whisper a mantra to myself, something inspiring, like "blessed be this miraculous morning," or "the world is your oyster." I make myself a healthy breakfast and go about my day, smiling to myself and feeling upbeat.

I am the perfect mother, a wonderful wife, the personification of calm. My house, of course, is sparkling clean. I always say the right thing when my children are upset; I never yell; I'm never impatient. My children do their chores without complaining and remain calm and cheerful throughout the day.

I breeze through the day while my house organizes itself around me, all by itself. I go to bed feeling I have changed the world in ways big and small.

My life wasn't always like this. There was a time when I was constantly tired. I thought I couldn't do it all, and I felt like a failure. I was sure I just couldn't win. But now I'm stronger and more confident than ever. I take whatever comes my way in stride, never even breaking a sweat. These days, people admire me and look to me for life advice and inspiration.

"How do you do it, Olga?" they ask me. I consider answering that I'm a natural. I wake up perfect every day and I just can't help it! But the truth is that I have full control over my destiny and have become the best person I can be thanks to an amazing little secret I discovered. What secret, you ask? *Niksen*, or the Dutch art of doing nothing.

Not Your Usual Wellness Guru

Did you believe that? No? Good.

The only truth to that story was the sound of chirping birds in the morning, and that's because my dear husband — after years of watching regular alarm clocks shock me awake — took pity on me and bought an alarm clock that sounds like birds singing. And while it's definitely an improvement over what could have just as well been used as a fire siren, my mornings are still traumatic. I have three children who I need to get out of bed and off to school by 8 a.m., preferably fed and dressed. By the time the school bus arrives, my sanity is usually hanging by a thread. But that's just the beginning; while my children are at school, I rarely find even a moment for myself.

Between all I have to do for my children, home, work,

(2)

husband — who works long hours — and the rest of my family and friends, I try to remember the last time I actually did absolutely nothing. And fail miserably.

I used to be so good at it. When I was little, I would sit on my bed or in my father's favorite armchair and stare at the patterns in the rug or out of a window, thinking of absolutely nothing. Sometimes my parents would ask me what I was doing and send me off to do chores or homework, but I had ample time to daydream. And it felt so good.

But now? As a mother of three, a wife, a writer, and a business owner, I always feel hurried and pressed for time. Sometimes it seems like I'm writing with one hand, caring for my children with the other, cooking dinner with my left leg, and cleaning the house with my right.

Of course, I'm aware that I have chosen this. I wanted this life. But acknowledging this fact doesn't make it easier. I, like so many others I know, am just . . . so . . . busy.

The last time I sat on my couch and simply did nothing was a few months ago when I actually collapsed onto it. It was the end of the school year and I was exhausted, sleep deprived, and unable to function, just like I usually am at that time of year. The only thing I felt capable of doing was lying on the coach and staring into space, which was how my husband found me when he got home from work.

(3)

It didn't occur to me at the time that collapsing like this was the only socially acceptable way to do nothing. "The attraction of illness lies in its capacity to redeem one of the greatest vices of our society: not doing anything," write management professors Carl Cederström and André Spicer in *The Wellness Syndrome*.

What Was Going On?

Something was happening, and I didn't like it at all. I was very tired and feeling overwhelmed, but I had no idea what to do about it. In my years of writing about parenting I noticed how stress was a huge factor in so many people's lives and that everyone was feeling as overwhelmed as I was. But it took a little article in an unknown magazine to make me realize that this was symptomatic of a much bigger problem that didn't affect only parents.

Two years ago, reporter Gebke Verhoeven published an article called "Niksen Is the New Mindfulness" in the Dutch magazine *Gezond Nu*. I loved the idea and remember thinking: *Cool, finally someone is telling me it's okay to do nothing. Now this is a wellness trend I can get behind.*

But immediately after that I wondered: How am I supposed to do nothing? Whenever I allow myself to sit down my house starts talking to me. "Do me, do me, do me," whispers the laundry in a totally unsexy way. Did I remind the children to do their homework, asks my conscience? And when I look around, I see books on the floor and dirty dishes on the kitchen counter. I know there is no food in the house, and I have zero idea what I am going to make for dinner. How can I just sit on the couch when

(4)

I feel compelled to get up and take care of the house and everyone who lives in it (except for myself, that is)? New tasks constantly materialize as if out of thin air. If I want to sit down, one of my children is bound to get sick or up pops an appointment I need to make or something else I am suddenly reminded I have to do. How on earth am I supposed to find time for this *niksen*?

Yet, after reading that article, a curiosity started to grow in me. What was this thing the Dutch called *niksen*? And why couldn't I do it just a little more? I started to research niksen extensively and discovered that simply doing nothing can be enormously beneficial, especially for those of us who, like me, feel overwhelmed by our responsibilities. Doing nothing, or niksen, really is worth it.

My curiosity led me to write a few articles on the subject. Then in May 2019 the *New York Times* published my story "The Case for Doing Nothing." After a few days, it had been shared hundreds of thousands of times. It became very clear that I had hit a nerve.

The whole world wanted to know about niksen. Media from around the globe were sending me emails and interview requests. Literary agents and publishers were asking to represent me. I was ready to dismiss it as much ado about nothing (literally), but there was something about niksen that seemed to appeal to people everywhere.

As I began to process and analyze the response that niksen was getting, I realized that people were fed up with wellness trends telling them they weren't doing enough

(5)

and should work harder at improving themselves. This is one of the reasons people relate to the concept. It's the easiest kind of wellness you could possibly imagine.

But another thing struck me: we simply don't know how to do niks. Though not doing anything — or doing nothing — may sound simple, it is actually anything but. In fact, if I had a penny for every time someone asked me how to do more niks I would probably be a millionaire by now. I realized that most of us need help learning how to stop being so busy. I have written this book hoping I can shed some light on how to do nothing, and so that people everywhere realize it's okay to sit on the couch and do a little niks.

What does it mean to do nothing anyway?

Many people have asked me, what does niksen mean? Do I do nothing when I browse Facebook? When I sit on my couch and worry about my children? When I'm thinking about an article I want to write? When I meditate? The answer is no. You might call those things nothing, but in reality, they are not. These things are not niksen. To do niks does not mean to work, to perform emotional labor, or to be mindful.

And while niksen might appear selfish, lazy, or boring at first glance, it is none of those things. On the contrary, if done right, niksen can be a service to the community.

Niksen has many benefits. After my research on the subject, I believe that doing nothing can ultimately make us more productive. By taking breaks during our daily work, we can become better employees, avoid burnout, and work more carefully and deliberately. Niksen is also great for our creativity because it gives time for our thoughts to wander, which results in insights that we may have not come up with otherwise.

But mostly, niksen is playful. It's fun. I wish everyone had the time to play, fool around, experiment, and try out new things. Then, after that is done, we want to be able to sit and contemplate the patterns on our rugs and slowly figure out what to do next.

Could I Be Wrong?

Critics, most of them Dutch, have accused me of pulling a trend out of thin air. I wish I had the power and the creativity to single-handedly start a worldwide trend, but the truth is, I don't. Have you even met me? I wear jeans and T-shirts every day; there is nothing trendy about me!

I believe, however, that I can offer a unique perspective on the local customs of the Netherlands, which I have been observing since I moved here ten years ago. As a writer and journalist, I have been a keen observer of this country and its inhabitants. The Dutch obviously have deep knowledge of their own culture, but sometimes it takes an outsider to shine the spotlight on a custom that may seem normal to the locals. I have come to see niksen as an example of this, so normal to the Dutch that they don't even notice it.

The criticism did make me wonder, however: Is niksen

(7)

really a Dutch thing? My first language is not Dutch, and I was not born in the Netherlands. Was it possible I misunderstood the origins of niksen? An American friend who lives here and is married to a Dutch man told me she doesn't know anyone who does it. Yet while there may be skepticism, all Dutch people I have spoken to about niksen immediately understood the term. At the very least, it is clear to the Dutch what the concept means, even if some claim they don't niks themselves.

I can tell you that *niksen* is a Dutch word, and its meaning is undisputed in the Netherlands. Words don't usually become part of a language without some concept or philosophy attached to them. I also see that the Dutch can struggle with niksen just like the rest of us. And I find that refreshing.

Whether knowingly or unknowingly, the Dutch have created circumstances for people to embrace niksen with more ease than many other cultures and countries. In my opinion, the Netherlands is a perfect place for niksen. Yet one of my favorite things about niksen is that, while it is a Dutch word, it doesn't belong to the Netherlands alone. In fact, as you will find out, many cultures have some concept of doing nothing.

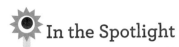

In the Spotlight

·······················

The Perks of Being an Outsider

I was born in Poland to a multicultural, multilingual family and have been living in the Netherlands for the last ten years. I grew up in Germany (where my husband is also from), and I have connections to France and the Netherlands, where my father and mother, respectively, spent part of their childhoods. I have grandparents and family in Ukraine, and I have Jewish roots too.

People don't always know what to do with me. "What are you?" they ask me. "How can we label you? What should we do with you?"

I'm an outsider wherever I go, and that can be hard. After all, we all want to belong.

And yet there are some benefits to being an outsider. No one knows this better than artist and writer Jenny Odell, author of *How to Do Nothing: Resisting the Attention Economy,* who is biracial herself. "Being an outsider can be helpful in finding unfamiliar perspectives on the supposedly familiar," she told me in an email. And I agree.

"As uncomfortable as it has been not being able to fit into any one category," she said, "this quality gives me a way not only of observing such categories from the outside, but of drawing connections across them that might not have occurred to me otherwise."

Outsiders often seem to be unsure of who they are,

(9)

but nothing could be further from the truth. In fact, a study by Hajo Adam showed that moving abroad can help people develop a clearer sense of self. Adam calls this "self-concept clarity" and defines it as the extent to which someone's understanding of himself or herself is "clearly and confidently defined, internally consistent, and temporally stable."

In *Range: Why Generalists Triumph in a Specialized World*, writer David Epstein argues that it is the range of experiences that many expats have that makes them successful. Instead of living one way, as the locals do, the outsider collects a wide breadth of experiences. Many find their career paths later in life and take detours getting there — both literal and metaphorical. They experiment with various jobs and in their personal lives.

For many outsiders, success comes not despite but because of their unique views and experiences.

The Problem with Wellness

Before we continue, I want to be clear about something: I'm no wellness guru, and this is no regular wellness book. In fact, I am just like many of you (maybe smaller: only five feet two inches, which is short by most standards and tiny in the Netherlands). And as much as I believe in niksen, I was a little skeptical about adding another book to the already overflowing wellness shelf.

My research, however, has convinced me that it's actually essential that I do. Most of us need to do a little more niks, and surprisingly, few of us know how to let go of our to-do lists. And while I don't claim to be an expert, I have researched niksen extensively for my articles and this book.

Still, it is with some apprehension that I am going to set about convincing you to bring niksen into your life. I have mostly succeeded in staying away from wellness and self-help books, with some exceptions. But I did fall for another genre of advice books: parenting. Ten years ago, when I first became a mother, I felt so pressured to be a good parent that I read everything I could find on the subject.

Interestingly, nothing I read made me more confident about my ability to parent. The opposite happened: I started to feel worse. There are similarities between parenting books and self-help books in that they both tend to talk at us (and not to us), with mild concern and a patronizing tone. Inevitably, the expert is intent on showing you how wrong your ways are, how much better your life could be. It took me a while before I realized the books weren't making me happier, just more insecure. When I saw this pattern, I stopped reading them. (My parenting skills have never been better.)

The irony of criticizing wellness trends in a wellness book does not escape me, but it is actually an important part of this book. I believe niksen is different from most wellness trends, and I'm sure that by the end of this book you'll agree with me. First of all, unlike other wellness trends, niksen doesn't ask you to change or improve yourself. Isn't that refreshing?

I'm sure many will agree that wellness trends can be harmful. If, for example, we expect healing crystals to cure cancer or vaginal steaming to balance our hormones (no, don't laugh — it's a thing popularized by Gwyneth Paltrow), we're setting ourselves up for disappointment and possibly even harm.

And by now wellness is everywhere. "Wellness has wormed itself into every aspect of our lives... It dictates the way we work and live, how we study, and how we have sex," write Carl Cederström and André Spicer in *The Wellness Syndrome*. They are not fans, likening wellness to an ideology that harms the vulnerable: "When health becomes an ideology, the failure to conform becomes a stigma." At the same time, it is accepted that "healthy bodies are productive bodies," and the same goes for happiness. It has become a social obligation to be happy and healthy, or else we become a burden on society.

The expectation is that we take responsibility for our happiness, says Paul Dolan, an economics professor and author of *Happy Ever After: Escaping the Myth of the Perfect Life*. The reality is that our quest for happiness is often devoid of even a drop of joy. It's all work, work, work. Dolan sees in this attitude a social narrative that "makes prescriptions about what people should want, think and feel." And it's not making us happier. I believe that in many cases wellness can be seen as part of a movement that increasingly pushes people to take matters into their own hands and look for alternatives to conventional treatments. This is partly a positive development, because while it's vital that we understand the various ways our lifestyle choices affect our health and well-being, they are more than just a private matter. A healthy diet is important, but it will not cure cancer. Solid and accessible health care and social security are essential. And wellness, in my opinion, risks shifting responsibilities from institutions, governments, and society in general onto individuals who are in need of help and support in times of struggle.

Some critics have agreed. In a review of Barbara Ehrenreich's book *Natural Causes: An Epidemic of Wellness, the Certainty of Dying, and Killing Ourselves to Live Longer* in the *New Republic*, Gabriel Winant describes wellness as "a coercive and exploitative obligation: a string of endless medical tests, drugs, wellness practices, and exercise fads that threaten to become the point of life rather than its sustenance."

In addition, wellness tells people, especially women, to constantly improve themselves. We have to work on ourselves, whether it's on our minds, our bodies, or our surroundings. Go to the gym, do yoga! Clean out your house! Work harder, because if you don't you are a loser and a quitter. "The pressure we put on people to be everything is

(13)

making most of us just feel like nothing," says Mary Widdicks, a psychologist, writer, and mother of three.

Then there's the fact that most wellness trends want you to believe that they are the ultimate solution for everyone and anyone. "If you jam yourself in someone else's model, that can get in the way of getting to these deeper values," counters Gretchen Rubin, a writer and podcaster who covers happiness and productivity in her books, such as *The Happiness Project* and *The Four Tendencies*. In short, you do you.

 ## In the Spotlight

Wellness Trends Around the World

In recent decades, wellness trends from all corners of the globe have come and gone, and I am sure there will be new ones in the future. Here are some of the most important or popular ones.

MINDFULNESS
Mindfulness, most frequently in the form of mindfulness meditation, has been around for at least 100 years, but its popularity exploded in the 1970s. While it originated from ancient Buddhist teachings, its ability to release symptoms of stress and anxiety helped make it a popular Western lifestyle practice. The general idea is

to restore your inner equilibrium by paying attention to your present state of mind and focusing on your breathing, watching your thoughts as they come, without judgment or shame. Practicing mindfulness can make you calmer and more engaged with yourself and other people.

ZEN

A similar philosophy is Zen. Japanese writer Naoko Yamamoto explains that "in Zen practice, you have to focus on now and try to forget about the past and future." According to an article on BBC Religion, through Zen practice people attempt to understand the very nature of life rather than relying on logical thought or language. And in this, Zen is very different from niksen or, as the aforementioned article puts it, "Zen is something a person does."

HYGGE, KOSELIG, GEMÜTLICHKEIT

In 2016, the world became fascinated with *hygge* (pronounced *hoo-gah* or *hyoo-guh*), an untranslatable Danish word that refers to spending time with friends in a pleasant, relaxed atmosphere and enjoying the simple things that life brings. In fact, this word proved to be so popular that it became a finalist for Oxford Dictionaries' Word of the Year in 2016.

(15)

Hygge is about sheltering from the harsh winter at home, covered in blankets and dressed in warm sweaters, preferably in a house decorated with furniture of Danish design. The Norwegian concept of *koselig* is very similar. The website *Life in Norway* describes it as follows: "More than anything else, koselig is a feeling: that of coziness, intimacy, warmth, happiness, being content. To achieve the feeling of koselig, you need koselig things. In darker months, cafés provide blankets on their outdoor chairs, and shops light their entrances with candles."

Another similar lifestyle philosophy is the German *Gemütlichkeit.* As the website *The Local* explains, "The word encompasses sensations of coziness, contentment, and warmth." The term can also be extended to refer to the sense of social acceptance and well-being.

KONMARI
Popularized by Marie Kondo in *The Life-Changing Magic of Tidying Up*, the KonMari method of house organizing and cleaning addressed people's need to declutter and their desire for a more minimalistic lifestyle. Suddenly everyone was downsizing and gazing at their belongings to see if they sparked joy and then throwing them away accordingly.

DÖSTÄDNING, OR SWEDISH DEATH CLEANING
This is KonMari's somewhat morbid cousin, which is cleaning out stuff before you die so that the people who

outlive you don't have to deal with it, thus saving them a lot of heartbreak. Margareta Magnusson, the author of a book on the topic, believes death cleaning is supposed to be hard but not sad. She advises starting with the easier objects, like whatever has been sitting in attics and garages, then moving on to more emotionally charged things.

A FEW OTHER TRENDY TRENDS

More recently the media has been abuzz with the Korean concept of *nunchi,* which involves being attuned to other people's emotions in order to build connection, trust, and harmony. To be great at nunchi — or, to have a quick nunchi — one needs tact, perceptiveness, and an understanding of complex social situations.

The Japanese concept of *ikigai,* a path to finding your life's purpose, has been called the secret to happiness, health, and a long, fulfilled life. Ikigai is the cross section of your values, the things you enjoy doing, and things you're good at.

So Why Do We Need Niksen?

With such a large variety of trends, philosophies, and quick-fix solutions, do we need yet another fad in our lives? I'm often asked this in interviews, and I am not surprised. After all, doing nothing hardly seems like a revolutionary idea. But as you'll discover, there is so much more to niksen than doing nothing. Much, much more. In this day and age, with everyone leading incredibly busy lives, refusing to run around like a headless chicken is nothing short of extraordinary. As you become comfortable with niksen, you will also become more comfortable with refusing to be so busy. Niksen will help you let go of some of that busyness instead of adding to it.

Yet busyness is only a part of the problem. There's also the constant pressure to perform that we feel in every area of life. We expect ourselves to give everything at work (never wasting time and always becoming more productive) and then go home to an immaculate and well-organized house (please let me know how to do that!), raise well-behaved and creative children, and have time to drive them to all sorts of stimulating sports and other activities while not ruining their lives. And let's not forget that we're expected to be supportive spouses or partners. And what about your health? Have you tried spirulina or kale? Have you been to the gym lately? Are you ready for your next marathon? And if these questions make you angry, then what about that mindfulness workshop to turn you into a calmer, kinder person?

We expect ourselves, as the Germans say, to be an *eierlegende Wollmilchsau:* a pig that gives milk, eggs, and wool, on top of meat. We strive to be everything, for everyone, at all times. Being a modern-day human is exhausting.

It is from this frame of mind, feeling we are not good enough, and in our quest for perfection that we then read about hygge or KonMari or whatever new trend is the flavor of the day. But what extra effort will this require from us? What will we have to *do*? What will we have to *buy*?

Niksen appeals to a desire for a simpler, more minimal lifestyle. Decluttering our lives has gained in popularity over the last years, and I don't believe the interest in niksen appeared out of the blue. The desire to do nothing may be as old as time. It has just been dormant. It's as though it didn't have a name and was therefore difficult to talk about. This changed when people discovered niksen—a word they could easily pronounce—and the conversation erupted.

I thought long and hard about the best way to use this word in English and in this book. "Engaging in niksen" sounded clunky, "to niksen" felt wrong. So, I decided to allow myself some space and creativity. Sometimes I'll use niksen as a noun, like, for example, in *the philosophy of niksen* or *the best thing about niksen.* Sometimes I'll say, "I love doing niks." But you'll also hear me say "niksening," and while it's not exactly grammatically correct, it works well in English. Finally, since I think there should be a word for a person who is doing nothing, I'll also use *nikseneer.*

What Will You Find in This Book?

Here, I'm going to share all that I've discovered since I began researching niksen, the Dutch art of doing nothing. I can tell you that niksen really does have the potential to change your life for the better. If we can stop being so busy, we can start being happier, more creative, more productive, and better at making decisions. This may not be easy, but I believe that it is possible.

Each chapter in this book will discuss a different aspect of the niksen way. Throughout each of the chapters you'll find what I call Spotlights with interesting facts or stories or expert opinions from people with experience living in the Netherlands or researchers who study some aspect of niksen. I'll draw from a wide range of disciplines, including, but not limited to, sociology, biology, psychology, history, and intercultural communication, as well as from my own personal experience. To my surprise, there wasn't much information available on doing nothing, so there was a lot I had to figure out on my own.

Each chapter will also end with three questions for you to niks on in your free time.

In the first chapter, you'll become familiar with the concept of niksen: what it is and what it isn't, the ways we approach doing nothing, and how we feel about it. Spoiler alert: we may not always be aware of it, but we all do it.

The second chapter is devoted to the Netherlands

and my observations of this small but densely populated country. You will become familiar with its peculiarities and ways of being. And, despite what some of its inhabitants may argue, you will see why this place is so perfect for niksen.

The third chapter explains where our constant busyness comes from and what it does to our health and social lives. Even though I'm a technology fan, I will tell you how screens are running our lives by taking up too much of our time. This chapter also goes into what stress does to our bodies and minds.

Chapter 4 then shows us the many ways niksen can positively affect our lives. This is where we find out how it makes us more productive, more creative, and more relaxed, and how it strengthens our decision-making skills.

The fifth chapter is practical: it teaches you how to introduce and embrace niksen in the most important areas of your life: work, home, and in public. It will be full of helpful advice on how to do more niks (if you are so inclined).

Chapter 6 talks about situations in which niksen doesn't work and addresses some of the criticism it has received. My conclusion is clear: Niksen can work for many of us but not all of us. If it's not for you, fret not. I have some advice on what to do instead.

(21)

And if you make it to the end of the book, I'll share whether I've managed to master the Dutch art of doing nothing myself or whether I have failed miserably. You can also expect some predictions for the future of work, leisure, and humanity at large. If you're wondering what such deliberations about the future have to do with niksen, the answer is: everything.

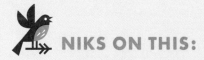
NIKS ON THIS:

• Do you feel busy and stressed out?

• When was the last time you did nothing at all?

• What do you feel when faced with the variety of wellness trends that are so popular right now?

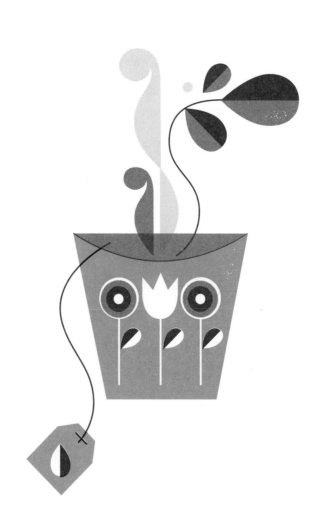

CHAPTER 1

What Is Niksen?

I'm sitting on my wonderfully comfortable brown couch. There is a mug of hot, steaming tea in my hands and I have my fingers laced around it, feeling the warmth. The mug is my favorite one, hand-painted in a floral pattern with other nature-inspired elements in green, brown, and shades of blue. The white Kindle that my husband got me last Christmas is probably lying next to me. In fact, I'm sure this is the case because I can't bear to part with my books for too long.

Cuddled into the couch, I'm feeling comfortable. My legs are bent under me and I'm leaning over one side with my left arm. Sometimes when my husband sees me folded up like this he asks, "So, are you Olga-ing around?" This position feels so natural for me that my husband named it after me.

Often when I'm seated like this, I'll be reading my book or editing an article I've printed. In both cases, it's pretty obvious what I'm doing: I'm either reading or working. Now, consider the following three scenarios.

1. I'm on my couch in the same position I've just described but I'm thinking about an article I want to pitch to an editor.
2. I'm still cuddled up on the couch, but in my head, I'm going through my day, planning dinner, mentally checking if the children have everything they need, or worrying about them.
3. I'm on the couch. I'm looking at my rug when my gaze moves toward the garden, and I notice the roses are still blooming despite the cold weather. My husband has put on some music and I'm listening to the singer's voice and the beat of the drums.

Which of these scenarios would you guess is niksen? Even if you don't know exactly what niksen is yet, I am sure you'll immediately recognize which of these three situations is an example of doing nothing.

Niksen: But How Do You Eat That?

When I studied at the University of Warsaw, I could have taken classes in Dutch, but this would have meant another year of school, and I had a boyfriend waiting for me in Germany. I was sure I would never need it, so I passed on that class. And yet here I am, having to learn this language anyway. Serves me right.

Some say Dutch is difficult, and that the pronunciation can be especially tricky. When I started learning the language, I went to the butcher and asked for five hundred grams (about one pound) of mincemeat. Or so I thought, because to my surprise, I arrived home with a tiny plastic bag filled with just a little bit of meat. Apparently, the way I said *vijf* (or five) sounded like *twee* (two). Go figure. I was too tired to go back for more and, luckily, I had lentils in my pantry. The result: almost-vegetarian meatballs. I'm nothing if not creative.

Besides being difficult, Dutch is also a fun, quirky language. "I would compare Dutch to a painting that uses a very wide palette of colors," says Marjan Simons, my Dutch teacher.

I'm particularly fond of the diminutives, such as *hondje, huisje,* or *bompje,* which mean "little dog," "little house," and "little tree," respectively. You just add *-je,* and the word becomes little. "We're the biggest people in the world, but our country is small. And everything we like becomes diminutive," says Simons.

I also love how you can turn everything into a verb. Playing tennis? No, *tennissen*! Paying with a debit card? No, *pinnen*! Having a drink (a *borrel*) and a plate of snacks with a group of friends? No, *borrelen*! Think of a word or expression, then turn it into a verb by adding *-en.* Doing nothing? No, niksen! It's brilliant, really. In my native Pol-

(27)

ish, when faced with something new, we say, "And how do you eat that?" So how do we eat niksen?

Do the Dutch Do Niks?

In Dutch, *niks* means "nothing," and it's just a small step from *niks* (which is a noun) to *niksen* (which is a verb). So niksen literally means nothing-ing. Marjan Simons offers an alternative explanation: niksen comes from *niks doen* (to do nothing), which is then abbreviated to *niksen*.

As I researched niksen, I learned of other Dutch words with similar meanings, such as *lanterfanten*. On her website BoekCoach (Book Coach), Dutch writer, editor, and entrepreneur Elise de Bres explains that *lanterfanten* is like niksen in that "you can just do as you please and there is no aim in whatever you do."

Another synonym is *luieren*. (You just try to pronounce all those vowels! I've been here for ten years and still can't manage.) In fact, the title of the Dutch edition of this book is *Niksen: De Dutch art of luieren*. At first, I thought this word meant being lazy, since *lui* is "lazy," but it also means "hanging out." Encyclo.nl, a Dutch online dictionary, defines it as "to consciously do nothing or not very much."

As a writer, linguist, and translator, I know that a language is a window into a culture. How is it possible, I wonder, that in a nation gifted with so many wonderful words for doing nothing, there are people who won't acknowledge that niksen is something they engage in from time to time, even if they were unaware of it?

Japanese writer Naoko Yamamoto has been living in the Netherlands for the last fifteen years, and she agrees that the Dutch are very good nikseners. "They can spend all day doing nothing on vacation, be it camping, lying around on the beach, sitting in the park, or simply staying at home. And on a sunny day lots of people sit around drinking beer or coffee on a terrace, just hanging around," she wrote to me in an email.

The Japanese, Yamamoto claims, are not great at niksen at all, but the idea does sound familiar to them. "Japanese people actually know that we have to have rest, so the concept of niksen is not very new, but showing them the way Dutch people niksen could be very inspiring to them," she says.

Is it possible that the Dutch themselves do not realize how much they already niks around? Sometimes it takes an outsider to see the truth.

In the Spotlight

....

Dutch People and Niksen

My friend Thessa Lageman, a writer living in The Hague, tells me she's very bad at niksen, and she is not the only one. "Many people can't do it. They would love to, but they feel the need to be useful." She also tells me that niksen was something the Dutch used to do quite easily before the internet existed.

Marjan Simons, my Dutch teacher, says she doesn't really see Dutch people niksening around very much. "We're very active. We have ice skating, hockey, we're very sporty. Otherwise, we're busy with hobbies and volunteer work," she says. When I ask her what Dutch people do to relax, she replies, "We do sports, we read a lot."

That's why Lageman thinks that niksen might be attractive to Dutch people "in this time of so many distractions." When I ask her whether the people I see sitting on benches in the park or lying on the beach are niksening, she hesitates before replying: "That's just part of the hiking or cycling trip, swimming, reading a book on the beach." Maybe this doesn't seem like niksen to the Dutch people, but it certainly feels like it to me.

Unlike Thessa, Anton de Jong considers himself an expert niksener. He defines niksen as sitting and soak-

(30)

ing up the sunlight. But he also believes that niksen can have both a positive and a negative meaning. It can mean either relaxing or being bored.

What Are We Doing When We're Niksening?

After determining the meaning of niksen in Dutch, I needed to find clarity on what niksen actually is. What are we doing when we're niksening? This question turned out to be much harder to answer than I had anticipated, as there wasn't much information available on niksen when I started researching it. Doing nothing might seem straightforward, but it isn't. Luckily, by digging deeper, I managed to get at some answers.

Carolien Hamming, a coach at CSR Centrum, a Dutch organization that brings together various experts in the battle against stress and burnout, says that niksen is "doing something without a purpose, like staring out of a window, hanging out, or listening to music."

Doing something without a purpose? That sounds great to me. You don't gaze out of the window to become a calmer, more relaxed human being, you do it just because. For the hell of it.

(31)

When I ask Manfred Kets de Vries, a renowned Dutch management scholar and psychoanalyst, what it means to do nothing, he says, "That's a very good question. You cannot do nothing. Because if you do nothing, you're dead."

It became clear early in my research that it's extremely difficult, maybe even impossible, to literally do nothing. Even when we sleep or rest, there are countless subconscious processes at work in our brains and bodies, most of which we're not even aware of. Our lungs are breathing, our hearts are pumping blood, our stomachs and intestines are digesting and secreting hormones. And that is a good thing, because I'm sure that if my breathing and my heart beating weren't regulated by my body, I'd forget to do them. "Oops, I forgot to breathe today," I'd sigh. "And can you please jump-start my heart while you're at it?"

We may not notice our hair and fingernails growing, but they are. Our brains are a constant flurry of activity as we lose old memories, cement others, and make new ones. We mull over problems and make plans for the future; we daydream. It's fascinating to see how much energy is involved in keeping a human being (even a sleeping human being) alive.

We can see human activity as a continuum. "You start at zero and you have zero energy expenditure and you're basically dead. Then at one, you are doing nothing at all and you're breathing and just sitting. And then you stand up, very slight physical activity, and then you walk, and then you run, that is vigorous physical activity," says Matthieu Boisgontier, a physical therapist who is fascinated with neuroscience and the author of a study showing that humans are a terribly lazy species.

Gretchen Rubin, author of *The Happiness Project,* has her own definition: "I would call it goofing off or puttering," she says. When I ask what that looks like to her, she offers this description: "I'm aimlessly knocking around my apartment or my neighborhood. I had to run an errand and now I'm just idling along. Sort of not in a hurry, not thinking about other errands. Just looking around. In my house, I'm looking at the mail, but only because it's randomly there." I find myself nodding along. "It's a Sunday morning kind of feeling. Just hanging out. It's loose, unstructured," she tells me, and I sigh because this sounds delightful.

As I collected expert opinions and definitions of niksen, I realized there is very little consensus on what it actually means. A number of experts I consulted associated it with the feeling of being bored. "The way I think about boredom is coming to a moment with no plan other than to be. Bringing your mind and your body to a place where you can literally just be idle," says Doreen Dodgen-Magee, a psychologist and the author of the book *Deviced!: Balancing Life and Technology in a Digital World.* When I ask for examples, she replies: "Like looking at clouds, just being able to look out of the window. Being with one's own thoughts without judgment, without literally going 'I have to do it as a mindfulness meditation' but just to be present." Reflecting on

(33)

that, I have to say that this sounds like niksen, not boredom.

As entertaining as these various definitions may be, a little more consensus on what doing nothing actually is would have been nice when writing this book. Instead, we each have our own definition. As artist and writer Jenny Odell admits, "Doing nothing might mean something different to everyone." Odell defines it as "finding even small interstitial spaces of non-goal-oriented activity—wherever one can get away with it. It's something you can do on the bus, waiting in line, and other in-between moments: just make the decision to observe as much as you can, without judgment, and with a willingness to be surprised."

 ## In the Spotlight

Doing Nothing Around the World

All around the world people have found ingenious ways to do nothing. Let's look at some examples to compare how people go about that. This list is not exhaustive; I am sure there are more that I don't know about.

DOLCE FAR NIENTE
Italy is famous for, among so many other things, great food and a relaxed approach to life. No wonder these

two can be combined to create one wonderful expression: *dolce far niente,* which literally means "sweet doing nothing." It's similar to the English phrase "sweet, sweet nothing" and the Dutch *lekker niksen,* as it describes doing nothing as delicious.

"It doesn't have a negative connotation. Because maybe *dolce far niente* is reading a book. It's an unproductive pleasant activity. Maybe you're watching a movie. It doesn't mean you're being lazy," says Silvia Bellezza, an assistant professor of marketing at Columbia Business School, who is Italian herself.

SIESTA
The idea of siesta is popular in many Mediterranean countries, especially in Spain and France. It's best known as time in the middle of the day when the weather is too hot to be outside and just right for a nap. But it's also a chunk of time that can be used for niksen.

SABBATH
The Jewish Sabbath, which starts at sunset on Friday and ends at sunset on Saturday, is a time for Jews to focus on prayer, family, and togetherness. Food is prepared before the Sabbath begins because work is prohibited during that time, as is electricity and any kind of screen, Rebecca Beck, a Hasidic Jewish woman living in Antwerp, tells me.

While idleness might be viewed with suspicion (hard work is appreciated in Jewish culture), Sabbath

(35)

is an important tradition and many Jews participate. And wouldn't we all benefit from a full day each week away from screens and full of quiet time and reflection?

MEET THE IDLERS

While the Dutch have niksen, the British have "the idler movement." In an interview with *Mother Jones*, the movement's founder, Tom Hodgkinson, says that an ideal world "would be full of people bicycling along the streets and whistling and raising their hats to each other, going for long walks in the countryside, and mucking about each day." If you ask me, that sounds a lot like the Netherlands.

WU-WEI

The Chinese concept of *wu-wei* (sometimes spelled *wuwei*) can be translated as "non-action." It stems from the Taoistic teachings of Lao Tzu, one of the most influential Chinese philosophers. "Some think it is pessimistic and passive. However, it can also be interpreted in a positive way," explains Amanda Hsiung Blodgett, a Mandarin teacher and blogger at *Miss Panda Chinese*. One way to interpret *wu-wei* is as "purposelessness." As you may remember, one of the definitions of niksen is "doing something without a purpose."

"LETTING YOUR INNER PIG DOG OUT" AND OTHER FUN EXPRESSIONS

Some cultures and countries frown on doing nothing. In one in particular, efficiency, excellence, hard work, and quality are held in high esteem: Germany.

One of my favorite expressions in German is *den inneren Schweinehund auslassen,* which can be translated very literally to "letting your inner pig dog out" (*Schweinehund* translates more correctly to "hog," but I like the idea of a pig dog). If you Google *innerer Schweinehund,* you will find loads of articles explaining how to fight your inner lazy beast, or *Schweinehund,* which in German is a derogatory term and even an insult.

Wictionary translates this expression as "shoulder devil" or "a weaker, lazy part of one's nature." While it's important to make good life choices, sometimes letting out your inner lazy beast isn't all that bad.

In other parts of the world, niksen is viewed more positively. For example, in Swahili, the word *starehe* means being "comfortably contented," like basking in the sun doing nothing.

Ilze Ievina, the author of the award-winning blog *Let the Journey Begin,* is originally from Latvia and tells me that in her language, *gurķoties* can be translated as "to pickle around" or "cucumbering around," which actually makes me laugh.

The ways people around the world approach doing

nothing is varied and incredibly creative. Whether pickling around or letting out your inner pig dog, there is no end to how we express our desire for time to wind down.

As you can see, niksen is not strange — it is a universal part of life.

What Niksen Is Not

In interviews about niksen I am rarely asked to define it beyond translating it from Dutch. It seems everyone immediately has some understanding of what it means, at least within the context of their own personal lives and circumstances. I think it's important to define precisely, however, as I have often found that people say they are doing nothing when they are certainly doing something, such as browsing Facebook or watching television. For this reason, I have found that the most effective way to define niksen is to first define what it is not.

Niksen Is Not Work
My father is a theoretical physicist. I'm a writer.

So much of what we do consists of sitting down with a piece of paper, thinking, and maybe writing something down. But mostly thinking. To an observer, this might look very similar to doing nothing. How can people know the difference, then?

They can't. Not until they ask or know the context in which we do our work.

But while it may *appear* that you are niksening at work sometimes, niksen is not work. Differentiating between these two can be hard, however, especially for creatives (like me).

"If you're a creative, you're never not working, because there are always problems you are trying to solve. We filter though the problems that we're processing and are at an impasse with," says productivity expert and acclaimed author Chris Bailey. Ideas, he believes, come not just from our external environment like a book that helps us solve the very problem we've been mulling over, but also from our own wandering mind. Thinking, therefore, is work; it is not niksen.

Niksen Is Not Emotional Labor
Fascinated by the idea that certain activities look like doing nothing but aren't, I tell Ruut Veenhoven, a well-known sociologist and a pioneer in studies of happiness, about the many moments I spend sitting on the couch being busy with a kind of work that can't be seen. I tell him about the worrying, planning, and making sure everyone in my family is happy. "You're ruminating. I wouldn't call that niksen," he tells me. I agree that the worrying isn't niksen, because it certainly doesn't feel like it, but I'm uncomfortable with calling this activity ruminating.

(39)

Journalist Gemma Hartley, author of the book *Fed Up: Women, Emotional Labor, and the Way Forward,* gives it a much better name: *emotional labor.* If I'm sitting on the couch and worrying whether I remembered to schedule my children's dentist appointment, I'm neither niksening nor ruminating. I'm performing emotional labor, the invisible mental load and emotional management required to keep those around us comfortable and happy. Emotional labor might at times look like niksen because it can be done while sitting on the couch.

"It's the mental calculations, the active empathy, the planning, tracking, and monitoring that happens inside our heads to keep everything running smoothly," Hartley explains. Personally, I felt both relief and exasperation when I learned that all this thinking, planning, and monitoring that I do has a name.

Classifying emotional labor as niksen would mean ignoring that this important work takes so much time, energy, and brain space for many women (because it's most commonly performed by women). It is thanks to emotional labor that so many lives run smoothly. Instead, I suggest we acknowledge the existence of emotional labor and help those tasked with it find more time for niksen.

Niksen Is Not Mindfulness

Though they may look similar, mindfulness is not niksen. While both share a quality of stillness, at their core these two activities are very, very different.

"I wouldn't consider meditation doing nothing," says Gretchen Rubin, who has experience with the practice. "I'm going into a posture, I'm focusing my mind, I'm setting out to do something even if there is no movement, but it's actually a very specific activity," she tells me. In my opinion, mindfulness and meditation actually seem like a lot of work: their effects can be calming, just not effortless. Recently, I found myself extremely annoyed by the hot summer weather and I was absolutely not going to relax and "be mindful" for that. So instead, I did something I don't usually do: I cleaned out my garage. I got rid of five big bags of junk, vacuumed the floor, and rearranged the items on the shelves so that everything could be found more easily.

I can't say I enjoyed it, but the deed was done quickly and efficiently. Why? Because I was not being mindful. I wasn't concentrating on what I was doing or my breath or my chakras, or even my body. I just tuned out the world and sang a song in my head and planned my day and thought pleasant thoughts that had nothing to do with the now.

Niksen might even be described as anti-mindfulness, as it doesn't require you to be aware of your body, your breath, the present moment, or your thoughts. Instead, you can use it for the opposite: you can use it to escape your head and just get lost for a while.

(41)

Niksen Is Not Laziness or Boredom

If you were caught lying around in the middle of the day, you might feel like you were being lazy, but a bit of niksening doesn't make you lazy at all.

My mom is a genetics professor and the most brilliant, talented, and ambitious person I know. I often watched her relax after a full day at work or between reviewing PhD theses and a next project, be it translating a patent or reviewing a science-themed book. As a result, I know that you can engage in niksen and not be lazy. As my writer friend Samara says, "No one would ever call me lazy. I work hard and I niks hard."

"We need to be careful how we talk about laziness because it has such negative connotations," Matthieu Boisgontier, the physical therapist, tells me.

And, while many of the experts I consulted about niksen specialize in boredom, there is a huge difference between these two things. Niksen is "doing nothing without a purpose," but boredom is defined as the experience of "wanting, but being unable to engage in a satisfying activity," according to a study by John Eastwood, a psychologist at the University of York. You do niks because you want to. When you're bored, you'd rather be doing something else. And that is exactly why I feel bored when I'm cleaning my house but never when I'm niksening.

*Niksen Isn't Reading Books, Watching
TV, or Browsing Social Media*

It's certainly tempting to call reading books, watching Netflix, or browsing social media "nothing." When someone asks us, "Hey, whatcha doin'?" that's often our reply: "Nothing!" But reading a book or watching Netflix certainly isn't niksen.

"People think they're taking a break a lot of the time, but they're not. They're just going from one distraction to the next. We go from a work context to just paying attention to our phones for ten minutes or so, and we stay distracted," says productivity expert Chris Bailey.

What we do online is not "nothing." It's working, networking, researching, or — like when I get stuck watching Tasty videos — procrastinating.

The same can be said of television. It can be entertaining, relaxing, a way to unwind or learn something new, but it's not niksen. This is an important distinction because I am not arguing that we should trade our fun (but not always terribly important) activities for niksen time. We use social media for a reason. We re-watch six entire seasons of *Glee* for a reason (or maybe that's just me). And all these reasons matter.

(43)

How We Talk About It

A first step toward understanding and appreciating the power of niksen is acknowledging our judgments about doing nothing and how we speak about it. Think about it: When do you use the word *nothing*? We tend to talk about doing nothing as though we're ashamed of it, especially in relation to work. "Oh, I'm doing nothing," we say when we think we should be working but are browsing Facebook instead. The word *nothing* often translates in some way to "unimportant." Or worse, "undesirable." Think of the child who tells us they've done "nothing" when there are obviously chocolate and crumbs all over the carpet and the special pralines you bought yourself are nowhere to be found.

"It seems quite a negative term, doesn't it? People say, 'I'm so lazy,' or people accuse other people of being lazy," reflects Sandi Mann, a British psychologist, bringing laziness back into the equation. "But it's not all bad because we sometimes say, 'I've had such a lazy morning' and that's seen as a good thing."

When my *New York Times* article on niksen was shared all over the internet, I had people near and far asking me for advice on how to find more niksen time. "I don't know," I would say, "sit down for five minutes, and just do it!" That wasn't very helpful, I'm afraid. Doing nothing doesn't come naturally to everyone.

"Just do it" bypasses important questions. Why can't we do nothing? Why is it so hard? Since then, I've reconsidered that particular piece of advice. Now, if asked I'd say, "Just do it, whenever you can. And don't worry if it's not possible for you or very difficult, or possible only for a short amount of time. Give it a try and see if it works for you. And remember, even a few minutes of niksen is enough."

One of the reasons niksen is so hard is because we feel ashamed when we engage in activities that are apparently less productive. We assign less value to activities that might be considered a waste of time, such as gazing out of the window, sitting still, or looking around the room, than we do to work. Activities that don't immediately yield results are therefore difficult for us to engage in. It's very hard for us to see value in doing nothing, mostly in light of all the things that don't get done while we do niks. Saying "just do it" is a little too easy when what is needed is a 180-degree change in perspective.

We need to start seeing niksen for what it is and for the amazing benefits it has to offer. Let's start to call a spade a spade, and niksen niksen. By extension, if we are browsing Facebook or chilling out with Netflix, let's call those what they are too and not say we're "doing nothing" when we're actually feeling guilty or thinking we should be doing something "better."

Niksen is not a random, unimportant activity. It has important, immediate, and long-lasting benefits. The Dutch say, "Doing nothing is good for nothing," but I beg to differ. Doing nothing is definitely not for nothing.

(45)

A New Perspective

By embracing niksen, people are finally allowing themselves to do less, not more. We're starting to realize we need to stop being so busy and slow down. And while niksen does require some work to find the time to wind down and look for little niksen pockets in our days, it does not require us to change anything about ourselves or our lives.

On the other hand, there are those of us who may want and need more time for nothing but feel they don't deserve it. These people can get caught in thoughts like "I'll do some niks after I've done two weeks of work that I'm behind on in one day, when my house is shipshape, my children in bed, and the five-course dinner has been prepared."

If this is you, please realize that you really don't need my permission to do niks (although just in case, you have it anyway). You are still a valuable human being if you take a little break.

And if you're still unconvinced, here are a few ways to rethink doing nothing so you will hopefully see how valuable niksen can be.

Taking a Break

"What's a break?" I ask Chris Bailey, the coach and productivity expert. "What I classify as a break is something that lets our mind wander at least a little bit. We're not 100 percent focused on something, and we don't have to regulate our attention in one way or another." While you might not always do nothing during your work break, the important element of both, to Bailey, is unfocused attention.

"When you're truly relaxed, you're usually not focused on something, and your mind has the chance to wander a little bit while you do something fun that you don't have to force yourself to focus on," he tells me. And his answer sounds exactly like niksen.

British psychologist Sandi Mann tells me that when she put people in a room where they were deprived of any sensory input and had nothing to distract themselves with, they struggled at first, but then eased into it. When they came out, they told Mann they considered it a mini-vacation.

Vacations are, of course, a great time for niksen, as long as there is no pressure put on the holiday. Destinations such as beaches, forests, or mountains are not just great places for hiking, swimming, and eating amazing food. They are also perfect backgrounds to doing niks. Relaxing on the beach and watching the waves hit the sand, like the Dutch so often do in the summer. Smelling pine trees in the forest and taking a quiet moment to relax before you start your picnic. Niksen is downtime, quiet time, finding a moment to unwind and relax, and maybe reflect a little.

(47)

Self-care

I am not a fan of the term *self-care* because caring for oneself shouldn't be just the individual's responsibility. In addition, it brings to mind images of expensive spa resorts and bubble baths. But since this term is currently so popular, I'm not opposed to using it if you want to do niks but feel guilty about not being productive. Self-care can mean taking a break from work or chores and giving yourself a moment to relax. In the words of writer Brianna Wiest, it means "building a life you don't want to escape from."

"I do see doing nothing as a potential form of self-care, but not in the commercialized form of it that we increasingly find. That's an important distinction for me, because it's so easy for ideas of self-care and self-help to simply fortify the boundaries of the commercial version of the self: something optimized and competitive," says artist and writer Jenny Odell.

Although self-care focuses on the self, it isn't selfish.

"I don't see 'doing nothing' as a way of protecting or merely comforting the self; rather, I see it as becoming open to one's community and surroundings, a readjustment of the self to her environment," adds Jenny Odell. Put like that, niksen could be seen as a service to the community and therefore not selfish at all.

Self-care is not always glamorous and set in luxury spas. In fact, it can be mind-numbing and terribly boring. Think of healthy eating, regular exercise, and keeping your home clean — all of this is self-care. So you can add to your self-care list a bit of niks and not feel bad about doing nothing; after all, I'm quite certain you don't feel bad about having a healthy meal. And though I've said that niksen is not work, I'll make an exception here: it is the work of self-care.

Daydreaming

I used to love doing it when I was a child. I would sit on the couch and do nothing. Well, it wasn't exactly nothing. I was imagining myself in the future, pondering the storyline of a novel I was reading, or simply thinking for the sheer pleasure of it. In short, I was daydreaming.

This was one of my favorite activities, and I still happily engage in it whenever I can. And I'm not alone. Our minds are not very good at remaining in the present, preferring instead to reminisce about the past or jump ahead to the future. According to one study, we spend almost 50 percent of our day daydreaming. And while not all of this daydreaming is done while we do nothing, some of it is.

Unlike mindfulness, and just like niksen, daydreaming requires no preparation, no training, and no special rooms or music. Instead, notice how good you already are at it. Start to notice when you're doing it and let yourself enjoy and savor it! Seeing niksen time in daydreaming can make it feel more accessible.

(**49**)

Wrapping It Up

There is a time and place for browsing Facebook, there is time for Netflix marathons, and there is time for niksen. We do these things for a reason. Let's own them all.

In this chapter, you learned what doing nothing is and what it isn't. You went on a tour of doing nothing around the world, and you thought about alternative ways to view niksen. You learned that people all over the world have words and concepts to describe doing nothing. But *niksen* is a Dutch word. Are you curious about the country and culture it comes from?

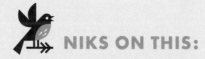

NIKS ON THIS:

• •

- What does niksen, or doing nothing, mean to you?

- Which of the suggested ways to think about it proved the most helpful?

- How does it feel to know that people all over the world have special words or periods for doing nothing?

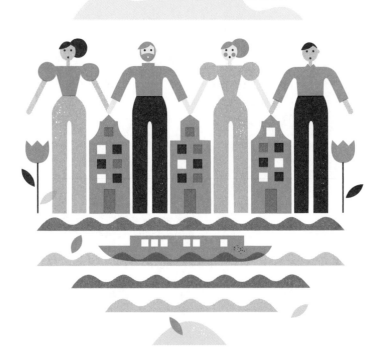

CHAPTER 2

What If the Dutch
Got It Right?

I'm sitting on my couch trying to recall the interior of my family apartment in Warsaw, Poland. It belonged to my mother's parents, who once lived in the Netherlands. Delft Blue plates decorate the walls, and there is a colorful Makkum tulip vase (which my father calls "the tulipanator") on the chest of drawers in my parents' bedroom. Even before I made the Netherlands my home, the Netherlands was, literally, in my home.

I have been living here for ten years, but my connection to this country goes further back than that. My grandfather was the Polish ambassador to the Netherlands in the 1950s and 60s, and he and his family lived in the Netherlands for eight years. He even wrote a book about his time here, *The ABC of Amsterdam,* which is a guide to living in the Netherlands, dealing with all aspects of life here from politics to culture.

Since I moved to the Netherlands, my mother, father, and brother have visited regularly. Often, we take tram 1 to the beach in Scheveningen, and when we pass by the Polish embassy, my mom can't resist telling us stories about the eight years of her childhood that she spent here. One of her favorite things to do is to go out for *poffertjes,* delicious tiny Dutch pancakes eaten with copious amounts of butter and powdered sugar.

How I Ended Up Here

I arrived in the Netherlands in 2009 with a six-week-old baby. No, I don't recommend moving at that time in your life, but the choice was to either live far away from my husband or just make the move.

At first, I found myself overwhelmed by motherhood, so my priority after arriving in the Netherlands was to simply survive. I needed to find food, clothes, toys, and the million little things you need in a household. To do this, I also needed to find out what these things were called in Dutch, which only added to my feelings of frustration. Only when my baby went to daycare at six months, like many Dutch kids, did I start to get a little more sleep, and I finally began to notice the country I had settled in. Some of what I saw felt familiar. Some things felt strange and new. Some I loved. Others, not so much.

We lived in Delft at the time, a small, quaint, and incredibly romantic little town close to The Hague. Delft was the capital of the newly independent Netherlands in the sixteenth century but is now mostly known for its blue-

and-white pottery. With beautiful old houses set along picturesque canals and grand churches, Delft looks like everything you've heard about the Netherlands squished into twenty-four square kilometers (9.2 square miles).

As I began to feel more like myself, I saw the beauty around me and realized that the Netherlands was indeed a very unique place. I took in the magnificent views of the canals and old houses, and noticed tall Dutch people bicycling all around me. My husband and I joined the locals in quaint cafés, where I soon learned to order *verse gemberthee,* or fresh ginger tea, usually served with a *speculaas* cookie and honey.

Small Country, Big People

The Netherlands has approximately 17 million inhabitants, of which 820,000 live in the capital, Amsterdam. This is pretty impressive given that the country stretches over only 42,508 square kilometers (16,412 square miles). Some people call it Holland, but this is actually incorrect. Holland refers to two of the country's twelve provinces: South Holland and North Holland. And it's in these two provinces where the most important cities, such as Amsterdam, The Hague, and Rotterdam, are located. To clarify this, the country is now officially rebranding as "the Netherlands."

By comparison, the United States is approximately 237 times bigger, while the United Kingdom is approximately six times bigger than the Netherlands. This country is so small that I tend to say that when you arrive by train or car and start saying, "We're now in the Kingdom of the Netherlands," you will have already crossed the border into Germany or Belgium by the time you finish the sentence. In addition to these two countries, it also has a maritime border with the UK, and is largely surrounded by water. It's no wonder that this element is often on Dutch people's minds.

In contrast to their tiny country, the Dutch (and especially Dutch men) are the tallest people in the world, averaging 183 centimeters (6 feet) tall. I, on the other hand, am 158 centimeters (5 feet 2 inches) tall. When I stand behind a Dutch person, I have to hope they won't move their arms or I'll get an elbow to the head — a situation I prefer to avoid.

Once my baby was in daycare and I started to really settle here, I learned to love the fact that I had the time to figure out what to do with myself. In a country with a faster pace of life, I would have probably become quickly overwhelmed and any creative endeavor would have been out of the question.

I love how safe and family friendly this country is. I love that I can walk or take the train, tram, or bus anywhere, be it to Delft, which I still visit as often as I can, or to The Hague (we now live in between these two cities). We take many day trips around the country and discover something new every time we go.

I soon noticed that the Dutch are . . . happy. Or maybe

happy isn't the right word. Neighbors greet one another on the streets, and people smile at me and my children when we're out and about. People rarely seem harried or stressed. While I could complain about the slow (and often bad) service here, my brother put it best when he said, "It's actually nice to be in a place where no one feels the need to hurry." In short, the Dutch seem satisfied with their lives in a calm and subdued way.

Several studies agree. Year after year the Netherlands scores highly on the World Happiness Index.

How is this possible? Did I die and wake up in heaven? Is it the tulip fields, the (partially) legal marijuana, or the cheese? (No, don't laugh, a study showed that cheese activates the same spots in your brain as opiates, although these kinds of claims must be taken with a great dose of skepticism.) It's certainly not the weather, so what is the secret of the Dutch?

Why the Dutch Are So Content

When I ask Gretchen Rubin, author of *The Happiness Project,* what people need to be happy, she immediately replies with "relationships." "We need deep enduring bonds, we need to be able to confide, we need to feel like we belong. We need to be able to get support, and just as important for happiness, give support to others," she explains. So whatever deepens and strengthens relationships makes people happier.

While healthy relationships make us happy, so does self-knowledge. "We have to know what our own interests are, our own values, our own temperament. It is only when we know ourselves that we can shape our lives in a way that will further our own happiness," Rubin says.

This makes me wonder. Could we find these two keys to happiness in the Netherlands: strong relationships and self-knowledge? It certainly appears that way.

I have heard many expats complain that it is hard to make friends with the Dutch.

"It's a tightly knit society where people have close friendship groups. They also often live in the same town or area their whole life," notes Ben Coates, a British writer and the author of the book *Why the Dutch Are Different: A Journey into the Hidden Heart of the Netherlands.*

The Dutch are supported by these strong relationships but also in other ways. When I ask Carolien Hamming of the stress research center CSR Centrum why the Dutch are so happy, she answers, "Social security. This is an enormous difference compared to the US, where people can end up on the streets."

Ap Dijksterhuis, a behavioral scientist who is also interested in the study of happiness, agrees. "What happy countries have in common is a stable democracy, a good social system, no poverty, no corruption, a government the people can trust, and some degree of wealth," he says. And all of that certainly applies to the Netherlands.

The World Happiness Report is mostly based on self-reporting and defines happiness as "how much you like the life you live," as sociologist Ruut Veenhoven explains. So, it has less to do with how people show their happiness, and more with how they feel about their lives. Therefore, the word *content* might be better suited to describe the Dutch than *happy.* "It's not so much about how you express happiness, because without that expression you can still be happy," Veenhoven explains. "We live in a prosperous and safe country. It's idealistic, with lots of freedom. People live a life that suits them." The Dutch know this and are content with it.

By contrast, Americans might be *too* focused on happiness, which actually makes them miserable. "Unhappy people think of happiness more than happy people do, just like patients are more concerned with health than non-patients. Research shows that happy people value happiness more and are more open to pleasurable experiences," Veenhoven says.

For me, it's really hard not to be happy in a country that's so stunningly beautiful. Sometimes I think living in the Netherlands is like living in a travel guidebook. And I'm not that far off when I say that. The Netherlands was picked as one of Lonely Planet's top ten best travel destinations for 2020. Everything you read about this country is true. The old houses along the canals? They're real. The tulip fields? They look exactly like they do in the photos. The windmills? Yes, also real. When my father and I visited the Netherlands in the mid-nineties, we tried to

(59)

count them, but there were just too many, so we gave up. But we still refer to windmills as "numbers" sometimes. I feel incredibly lucky to live here.

If this doesn't make you want to move to the Netherlands, I don't know what will.

 ## In the Spotlight

The Dunes, My Favorite Spot in the Netherlands

It's hard to overlook the dunes when you live in The Hague. After all, the city has 11 kilometers (6.8 miles) of coast. The dunes quickly became my favorite place to be in the whole country. Out of the 1,500 species of wild plants and flowers growing in the Netherlands, half can be found in various dune areas.

The dunes are absolutely stunning in every season, with yellow, white, and pink flowers growing in the spring and summer, and green, brown, and dark red mosses and grasses taking over during fall and winter. I love hiking through them with my family and taking in the changes in colors and temperatures over the seasons.

I have a fun little theory about why I love the dunes so much, and it has to do with the savannah hypothesis. Humans learned to walk on two legs when they moved from the forest to the savannah, and even though we have since moved to cities, we may still have a soft spot for that kind of landscape.

In fact, when people in a study were shown photos of various landscapes and asked which they liked best, the pictures of savannahs won hands down. Savannahs are typically flat, while dunes are hilly, but the dunes have a similar combination of shrubs and uniform grasses and are also inhabited by big grazing animals like sheep, Highlander cows, Konik horses, and even wisent, the European bison!

In a study performed by Columbia University psychologist Shigehiro Oishi, introverts preferred mountains, while their more outgoing counterparts tended toward wide-open plains. So, no wonder I love the dunes so much. They're the closest you can get to a mountain in such a flat country.

Happy and Healthy

The Netherlands is a nation of healthy people, with both a high life expectancy and high quality of life. The Oxfam Good Enough to Eat study ranked the Netherlands first in a variety of categories: enough food to eat, food accessibility, food quality, and health. The Netherlands has the best access to fruit and vegetables of the 125 countries it studied, which means that the Dutch can afford to buy fresh produce even if they don't have a lot of money.

Interestingly, another study by Euromonitor showed

(61)

that the Netherlands is one of the world's most sugar- and fat-crazy countries. The Dutch like to indulge sometimes and are not fans of depriving themselves. Meals are often served with French fries, and Dutch children eat *hagelslag,* or chocolate sprinkles, on slices of fluffy white bread for breakfast.

Dutch people are unlikely to be obese, so these treats have a place in a diet that's healthy overall. The Dutch enjoy snacks responsibly; some favorites are *bitterballen,* tiny fried croquettes, and *stroopwafels,* delicious syrupy cookies that have recently become a favorite snack for American professional basketball players. Many tasty delicacies are seasonal. *Oliebollen,* for instance, which are the Dutch take on the doughnut (and which translates to "oil balls"), are sold only from November 'til January.

Speaking of food, I love how the Dutch describe everything, not just their food, as *lekker,* or "delicious." Sleep can be lekker. Being warm can be lekker. Dancing? Definitely lekker. Calm and relaxation? Yum. Just yum. And to a Dutch person, even busyness is delicious, as they sometimes say, *Lekker druk!*

Which brings me to niksen. You can say *lekker niksen* because doing nothing is delicious too. This is a common expression in Dutch and is like the English phrase "sweet, sweet nothing," which expresses some of the same sentiment.

A country that has no issues with a bit of indulging, and that tends to call many things delicious, can easily give birth to niksen.

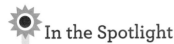

In the Spotlight

. . . .

Dutch Food

I met Li Bruno-Clarke through a group devoted to help-ing expats in the Netherlands find the ingredients they need to make food from their own country.

Li says: "I landed in the Netherlands with two suit-cases and a lot of nerve. I was recently divorced, on the edge of forty, with no job lined up but a whole lot of American can-do attitude. That whole move has proven to be the craziest and best decision of my entire life. As a food lover it was all so glamourous. I ate my weight in *oude Amsterdamse kaas* and *bitterballen*. Plus the wine from France and chocolate from Belgium because they were right over there!

"The hardest thing for me was actually lunchtime. I was used to 'dining al desko' — having lunch at my desk and getting a bit more work in. That does not work here at all. You are expected to go to lunch, and you are ex-pected to engage in conversations with your colleagues — mostly in Dutch. You may not ever get used to having milk or orange juice with your sandwich, but you will find out more about everyday life in your adopted new homeland."

(63)

Cultural Traits That Make the Dutch Happy

Pillarization

A typical trait of the Dutch is the so-called *verzuiling,* or "pillarization." "Some countries are a bit of a melting pot; they mix everything up and try to even out their differences. They try to make sure that everyone adopts the same values. But in the Netherlands, especially in the past, the tendency was to separate," explains Ben Coates, author of *How the Dutch Are Different.* As a result, "Catholics and Protestants have their own separate schools, hospitals, and universities."

Although pillarization is disappearing, the idea remains: to each their own, or in other words, live and let live.

"That probably feeds into the fact that people have the right to stand up and say what they think. And that's one of the great strengths of the Netherlands. It's probably why they're so tolerant and successful. Everyone has a right to be heard and have an opinion and have that opinion valued, even the children," continues Coates.

Just Be Normal

When the American women's soccer team won the World Cup, their public displays of joy did not go unnoticed. Megan Rapinoe especially was celebrated as the star of the tournament. The team's joy was a pleasure to watch, but not for everyone. "When you see the American ladies, after the third goal they're all *woohoo!* That's not Dutch," notes Catharina Haverkamp, an actress turned parenting expert and coach based in Amsterdam.

In the Netherlands, such outbursts of emotion are seen as weird at the very least and to some extent even insincere or rude. "We don't have to be happy all the time. That's not nice for the others. For us it is important to be a little humble," says Haverkamp.

This touches on something that's so ingrained in Dutch mentality that it has several expressions dedicated to it. The Dutch say, *Doe maar gewoon, dan ben je al gek genoeg,* or "just be normal, that's crazy enough." This doesn't mean that everyone must speak and behave the same way, but that excessive acts or emotional outbursts are frowned upon, and not boasting too much about achievements is encouraged. The belief is that actions speak for themselves.

Equality

When it comes to hierarchy in the workplace, organizations are flat, and the distance between employees and management is very small. Decisions are made by consensus, and everyone is expected to contribute, sometimes even people who have nothing or very little to do with the decision at hand.

This consensus gathering is called *polderen,* and it is a central part of Dutch democracy too. There are more than twenty political parties, and each time a government is formed there needs to be a majority coalition between many, small parties. Politics in the Netherlands is very much a matter of finding common ground and compromises.

 ## In the Spotlight

Comparing Dutch and Japanese Working Cultures

I met Japanese writer Naoko Yamamoto after I read an interview with her in *Business Insider* and I immediately reached out. I was fascinated by how niksen resonated in other countries and was curious to see how the Japanese working culture differs from the Dutch one.

Naoko says: "Firstly, there is a clear hierarchy in Japanese companies, and the decision-making process is much more complicated. We need lots of consensus to make a decision and the process takes a long time. In Japan, plans are made very carefully and perfectly.

"In the Netherlands, the relationship between the boss and his or her subordinates is defined by the fact that the hierarchy is quite flat. The decision-making process is much simpler and speedier. But sometimes decisions are made too fast and too carelessly, and they tend to fail more too.

(66)

"I think the hierarchy system and long decision-making process make Japanese work culture more difficult and stressful. We work unnecessarily long hours. After such a long process with perfect planning, we are also afraid of failure, of making mistakes. If we could work more like Dutch people, we would probably have more time for niksen.

"The education system also makes niksen difficult for us. First of all, we have lots of homework during summer holidays. I think this is why Japanese people are not good at niksen even during their holidays! Second, we are told to do things carefully and perfectly. We aim for perfection rather than fun. This forms our characters and affects how we can enjoy relaxing in life. Japanese education has to be changed.

"In my opinion, a kind of self-autonomy is needed for niksen. You have to take control of your life and say no to overwork. We need to learn to decide for ourselves that we want to rest and live our lives. We need to learn to think about ourselves!"

Children are also taught to share their opinions in schools, especially during the *kringtijd,* an activity in which they sit in a circle and everyone gets the chance to talk about their day. The circle is also the preferred seating arrangement for birthday parties in the Netherlands. The blogger Stuart Billinghurst calls this "the Dutch circle party" on his blog, *Invading Holland*. Simon Woolcot, a blogger known as the Amsterdam Shallow Man, goes even further and jokingly describes this as "the Dutch circle of death."

Another interesting thing about birthday parties here is that visitors are expected to congratulate everyone, not just the birthday boy or girl. This shows once again that equality is greatly valued here, and every guest is equally important.

There are some paradoxes that come with the equality, the contentedness, and the "just be normal" attitude. On one hand, individualism is appreciated, and you can love whomever you want, regardless of gender, age, or quirkiness, and no one will bat an eye. On the other hand, there is a strong expectation to conform. Ben Coates puts it well: "Yeah. You have to fit in. To be gay is completely fine and a man married to another man, that's fine. But if you put your trash out in the wrong container or on a wrong day, that is a major social scandal."

How does this work? Ruut Veenhoven explains: "Individualism goes together with egalitarianism in the Netherlands . . . This culture prefers cooperation over conformity to the directions of bossy people." In fact, the Dutch tendency to be normal—*doe maar normaal*—isn't really about conformity all. It isn't a result of social pressure, but rather a willingness and a desire to communicate and reach consensus.

Why Dutch Kids Are Happy

Not only are Dutch adults some of the world's happiest people, they are also raising the world's happiest kids. One reason is that the Dutch have a strong support network in place to help with their children through daycare, government-funded child support, and paid maternity leave.

But there is also something about the way the Dutch approach parenting. The sternest behavior I have seen from a parent was when her child was crying and she told him, "I want you to stop crying. That's not *gezellig*." (*Gezellig* is untranslatable but it means something like "cozy." You'll find a more detailed explanation later in this chapter.)

Instead of yelling, Dutch parents typically explain the reasons for their behavior, and ask their children questions. Kids are not rude, but they are active and assertive, and they are used to being heard and involved.

When children are newborns, Dutch parents create a calm, stable environment for them. This includes introducing strict routines and focusing on family time (activities for the whole family) rather than me-time (one-on-one time spent with a parent). A study comparing how American and Dutch parents interact with their children showed that stable surroundings make Dutch babies calmer and more relaxed than American babies, who are engaged with and played with more often.

"Dutch people consider childhood to be a very important time. They have quite romantic ideas about childhood. Be in nature, go outside, be free, explore your life.

And these are some things that make children in Holland happy," says Dutch parenting expert Catharina Haverkamp.

In the Netherlands, fathers play an important part in raising children. While they don't have as much parental leave as dads in Sweden, where fathers receive ninety days of leave, Dutch fathers are still very involved in the care of their children, starting at a very young age. Imagine my shock when I found myself the only mother on a playground in Delft; I was surrounded by fathers, and needless to say, I loved it.

Many men work one day a week less so they can be with their children. This is informally called *papadag,* or "daddy day," and formally, *ouderschapsverlof,* or "parental leave." A day off like this isn't possible for all fathers, but it allows many men to spend more time with their families and gives them time for not just parenting but also house chores, hobbies, and leisure activities.

Reading and interviewing experts about parenting here exposed another typically Dutch trait. The love of routine is expressed in the three R's of Dutch parenting: *rust, regelmaat,* and *reinheid,* which mean "calm," "regularity," and "cleanliness." The Dutch consider these to be very important values when it comes to raising children.

"The Dutch love to eat dinner at six. I think many families don't eat in front of the television. They eat at the table. It's their daily meeting point," explains Catharina Haverkamp.

Parenting in the Netherlands is certainly more hands-off than in the US and the UK, as well as in many other countries. When I ask Michele Hutchison, a British writer and editor who coauthored the book *The Happiest Kids in the World: Bringing Up Children the Dutch Way,* what she thinks of Dutch parenting, she says, "If you talk to Americans, they're set on giving their kids the best start, getting them into the best university, and having them involved in extracurricular activities." But in the Netherlands, life for children is more laid-back. Michele's children, now teenagers, didn't have any homework until they started secondary school, and there was less pressure on them to succeed and come home with good grades or trophies.

 ## In the Spotlight

Dutch Parenting

Amanda van Mulligen has been an expat here for a long, long time.

She says: "My three sons were all born in the Netherlands. They're being raised with a tinge of whatever Britishness I can instill, but they are clearly Dutch. The country I now call home has influenced my parenting journey. It's different to how parenting would have been had I stayed in Britain.

"For starters, independence is important early on for the Dutch. Many children make their own way to and from their primary school, usually on their bikes. And

(71)

my sons are no exception. My twelve-year-old cycles forty minutes each way to his secondary school. The British part of me fretted when he started his new school, and it felt un-Dutch of me. However, other Dutch mothers assured me that they worried too, but you set rules, send them off into the world, and hope for the best. It's how kids develop into responsible, happy adults.

"What I love most about living in the Netherlands with children is the emphasis on play. My primary school–age sons have virtually no homework. That means they have ample time to roam through our village with their friends. They play cops and robbers with walkie-talkies or play football or ride their bikes. Whatever the weather. They wander home in time for their dinner.

"Most evenings we eat together as a family. The Dutch work-life balance culture facilitates that. It's not something I grew up with because of my father's working hours, and I know that's an alien idea for my friends back in England.

"The one thing I haven't embraced from Dutch parenting? *Hagelslag* (chocolate sprinkles) for breakfast. My kids eat cereal for their first meal of the day."

Why Dutch Women Are Happy

The book *Dutch Women Don't Get Depressed* by science journalist Ellen de Bruin argues that Dutch women are the happiest in the world. While the title was initially meant as a parody of books like *French Women Don't Get Fat,* de Bruin found as she talked to all sorts of experts, including historians, psychologists, expats, and others, that Dutch women are indeed happy. According to de Bruin, this has to do with high levels of personal freedom.

The Dutch, as an individualistic nation, have a lot of choices about how to live their lives, and women are no exception. They can marry whomever, whenever they want or not get married at all. Moreover, Dutch women don't feel pressured to adhere to the rules of authorities, and this has a positive effect on their feelings of happiness.

Maybe most important, though, is the fact that in the Netherlands, there is no expectation of a perfect appearance. Women dress for comfort and practicality rather than to stun the onlooker. And dressed in their jeans and sneakers, they are direct and outspoken, with a strong sense of personal empowerment.

Last but not least, Dutch women rarely experience the burdens felt by women in other countries who are required to take care of not just their children but also their aging parents. Most Dutch people will agree that caring for children is the parents' responsibility but caring for the elderly is a job for the government. State-run homes for the elderly are a fact of life and accessible for all. The Dutch have a word to describe the nuclear family—*gezin* —as opposed to *familie,* which is the whole family, and the two are viewed as different and separate family units with different priorities.

Although fathers are involved, mothers reduce their

(73)

working hours more than fathers in order to care for their children. This might also be a contributing factor in their high levels of happiness. Many women here work part-time whether they have children or not, and this has been linked in several studies to increased feelings of happiness. When women have time for professional activities as well as their families and hobbies, they generally feel happier. The Netherlands is a great place for this kind of work-life balance, as it's practically the norm here.

 ## In the Spotlight

The Six Dimensions of Culture

In the late 1960s and early 1970s, Dutch researcher Geert Hofstede worked with IBM offices around the world to find out what employees valued in different countries. His findings resulted in the six dimensions (or 6-D) model of culture. Let's see what they are and how the Netherlands compares to other countries according to Hofstede Insights, an organization that helps companies bring cultural awareness into their business dealings.

1. Power Distance
Hofstede Insights defines this as "the extent to which the less powerful members of institutions and organizations within a country expect and accept that power is distributed unequally." The Dutch score very low (38 on

a scale from 0 to 100) on this dimension, reflecting their value for things like being independent, having equal rights for everyone, decentralized power, and direct communication.

2. Individualism

This is defined as "the degree of interdependence a society maintains among its members." The Netherlands scored 80 points on this dimension, making it one of the most individualistic countries in the world. Family members are expected to care for themselves and their closest kin. Hiring and promotion decisions are supposed to be based on merit rather than connections.

3. Masculinity

This dimension doesn't refer to gender roles but rather tries to define whether a society prefers competition, winning, and success (masculine qualities) or cooperation, caring for others, and quality of life (feminine). "The fundamental issue here is what motivates people, wanting to be the best (Masculine) or liking what you do (Feminine)."

The Dutch score 14 out of 100, making it a very feminine society. This means that things like consensus, support, work-life balance, and solidarity are valued more than success and competition.

4. Uncertainty Avoidance

This dimension measures "the extent to which the members of a culture feel threatened by ambiguous or unknown situations and have created beliefs and institutions that try to avoid these."

With a score of 53, the Dutch score in the middle, with a slight preference on the side of avoiding uncertainty. This might mean that they have strict codes of belief and behavior. People also feel the need to be busy and not waste their time, while in countries with low uncertainty avoidance the opposite is true.

5. Long-term Orientation

This dimension is pretty much self-explanatory, but here's a definition anyway: "How every society has to maintain some links with its own past while dealing with the challenges of the present and future."

The Netherlands score a rather high 67 out of 100, which reflects that its people are incredibly pragmatic. They also like to prepare for the future, be thrifty and careful with money, and tend to be very adaptable.

6. Indulgence

With this dimension, researchers want to understand how important it is for a culture to "try to control their desires and impulses." Cultures are either indulgent or restrained. You might think that the thrifty, pragmatic Dutch would be a restrained culture, but they score very highly on the indulgence dimension. Just visit the Netherlands during Carnival, King's Day, or a big soccer match, and you'll understand immediately.

Why the Netherlands Is Perfect for Niksen

While many Dutch people have told me that they don't feel they have time to do niks, I beg to differ. If there is a place that makes doing nothing easy, it's the Netherlands. With a generous social support system, short workweeks, and a lot of time off, this country is almost a niksen paradise. I'll admit that the Dutch are busier and more stressed out than ever, but the Dutch culture allows people to niksen. You want proof? I have plenty.

Punctuality and Agendas

When the nurse at the baby consultation clinic asked, "When do your children sleep?" I replied, still bedazzled by my newborn, with this gem of an answer, "When they're tired."

Suffice to say that I do not own an agenda. An item like that can be lost, and I don't always carry a handbag, so I wouldn't know where to put it. And while I could use my mobile phone, I spend so much time online that I'd rather not have another reason to look at a screen.

Instead, I use a magnetic board that is on the wall behind my desk that I attach Post-it Notes to, then I take them down when I no longer need them. That way I don't become overwhelmed by appointments and I manage not to forget them.

My friends living in the Netherlands often complain how hard it is to spontaneously meet with the Dutch. Their agendas are often filled to the brim with professional as well as social appointments. This can be a challenge for outsiders looking to mingle and socialize, especially for those of us who come from a culture where you can say, "Oh sure, I'm coming over in about five seconds."

The Dutch don't do anything without consulting their agendas first. And this is great for niksen, because if they can use their agendas to schedule appointments, they can also jot down niksen time on those same pages.

The What of What? On Gezelligheid

According to Geert Hofstede's six dimensions of culture model, the Dutch typically score high on individualism. They also value pleasure, indulgence, and enjoying themselves.

These qualities and values come together in the Dutch concept of *gezelligheid*. This comes from *gezellig*, which is an untranslatable word you may have even heard of; it's right up there with the Danish *hygge*, German *Gemütlich*, and Portuguese *saudade*. While it can be roughly translated as "quaint," "having a nice atmosphere," or "nice," it's not entirely any of these things. It's uniquely Dutch and can be applied to all sorts of situations, from a cozy family evening, to a dinner for two, to a big boisterous party.

(78)

My grandfather, the Polish ambassador to the Netherlands, defined *gezelligheid* as "everything that warms the heart and makes you smile." I think this is my favorite definition of this word. And I think niksen can be seen as *gezellig* at times as well!

Critical Thinking

The Dutch are critical thinkers, and they are unlikely to unquestioningly accept a new trend. This could be why niksen wasn't considered a trend in the Netherlands before American media picked up on it. And that's a good thing. Mindlessly embracing any hype that appears on the horizon was never my thing either. I am, after all, the daughter of two scientists, and I usually poke fun at wellness trends (too strict! too much work! no time for that!).

Egbert Schram, a Dutch national living in Finland who works for Hofstede Insights, tells me that in the Netherlands people almost automatically keep a feedback loop running, especially when there are multiple perspectives. "This means that it's perfectly acceptable for a Dutch person to switch their point of view on something the moment new data becomes available."

One great advantage of Dutch critical thinking skills is that they result in a fabulous sense of humor! This became visible in the responses to a *New York Times* article about the Dutch tradition of dropping teenage children in the forest in the middle of the night and letting them find their way back to a camp. While this might seem negligent to many readers, the truth is that the kids walk in groups, are never alone, and since the Netherlands is such a small country, no one can really get lost. Moreover, this also points to differences between American and Dutch parenting: independence is a big part of being a Dutch child. Americans were somewhat shocked by the article.

(79)

The Dutch were not having it, and the comments on Twitter were hilarious and brilliant too:

"True. It's part of our beautiful Dutch culture. That's why I gave birth 8 times in the forest. 3 of them eventually made it home, the strong and independent ones," wrote one Dutchie.

"I'm not even sure if the family I eventually found is my real family. But we made it work," wrote another. "OMG THEY'RE SUPPOSED TO COME BACK?" wrote yet another one, proving once and for all that the Dutch are a funny group of people.

Catharina Haverkamp agrees. "I think that's because the Dutch are optimistic and have a sense of humor, and that helps to make things feel less serious. It's the way we help each other. Make a little joke. Make things less important."

Directness

One day, I was trying to breastfeed my middle daughter at the local *kinderboerderij,* or "petting zoo," when a woman sat down next to me and said, "I think it's really important that you breastfeed." I was so stunned that I couldn't think of a reply, especially with one breast out of my bra and a fussy baby to feed. Why did this total stranger feel she needed to share her opinion on the way I was feeding my baby? But there she was, acting like throwing advice at someone you don't know is a totally normal thing to do.

This can be perplexing to people from other cultures in

which a sense of politeness and good manners would prevent someone from even thinking about such a comment. And so the Dutch often come across as rude. But from the Dutch perspective, there is nothing rude about this at all. It's simply communication.

"The Dutch don't think of this as rude. They think of it as honest. And what I, a British person, think of as polite or diplomatic, Dutch people would say is pointlessly lying or being dishonest," explains Ben Coates.

I must admit that I initially found this trait upsetting. But I have learned to appreciate it and can see it has advantages. It allows parties to clear the air very quickly. The Dutch cut through the fluff and give you facts — or their opinion. If you get this directness right, it can be very, very effective.

Openness and Tolerance

Also characteristic of the people of the Netherlands is their openness. Just take a look at Dutch houses and their huge windows. You can stare into everyone's home as you walk down the street. Some people don't even have blinds or curtains and are practically inviting you to take a peek. While this says, "I have nothing to hide" (and also, "I buy all my furniture at IKEA"), you are actually expected *not* to gaze into people's homes just because you can.

Still, openness is a fact of life here, and in this country where literally nothing is taboo, people rarely feel the need to hide anything about themselves. According to the

Dutch, there is nothing that can't (or shouldn't) be talked about. They call this *bespreekbaarheid,* or "speakability," which means they are not afraid to openly discuss difficult or uncomfortable topics.

While this can be hard to wrap my head around at times, I've come to believe that *bespreekbaarheid* is a good thing. Not speaking about our problems can lead to issues by itself, such as, among other things, depression, anxiety, and anger. The fact that the Dutch are willing to talk instead of tamping things down probably contributes to their general happiness. So, while it may feel odd, rude, or surprising to outsiders and foreigners, there is freedom to be found in saying what you think and not hiding anything.

By extension, in the Netherlands, where people don't feel the need to hide anything, if someone were going to do a bit of niksen, they wouldn't need to think of an excuse for doing nothing. It would be perfectly acceptable to say, *ik zit te niksen,* or "I'm niksen-ing." There is a lot we can learn from the Dutch, and not being ashamed is one of these things.

(82) The Dutch: Happy or Depressed?

A 2013 study surprised many people when it concluded that the Netherlands was the world's most depressed nation.

I decided to ask Ruut Veenhoven what he thinks about this. "Nonsense" is his reaction. And he goes on: "The treatment for depression is not equal everywhere. Treatment requires recognition." So a country that recognizes and treats depression appears to have more depressed people than a nation where it isn't being recognized and treated.

I also checked in with Carolien Hamming, and her response to the study is this: "How do you measure that? Do you go to the doctor? How does society see it? There is this contrast, we're high in happiness and high in depression."

And her comments make sense. People are actually more likely to be depressed in WEIRD countries, that is, Western, educated, industrialized, rich, and democratic. According to one hypothesis, it's the sharp contrast between how happy everyone else is and how a depressed person is feeling that makes living in a happy country so jarring. This is known as the dark contrast paradox.

Moreover, people in Protestant countries (like the Netherlands) tend to be more depressed than those in Catholic countries — but only if you're already prone to depression. One theory is that the individualistic tendencies of Protestantism, paired with the belief that your life has been predetermined before birth, make depressed people feel even worse.

That said, in the Netherlands a strong support system makes up for the challenges of an individualistic society while simultaneously encouraging self-determination and a chance to create a life that fits your character, values, and beliefs.

As Carolien Hamming concludes, "We have it good as a nation."

Wrapping It Up

In this chapter you learned why the Netherlands consistently shows up as one of the happiest nations on Earth and what makes it such a great place for niksen.

The Netherlands is such a perfect place for doing nothing. Dutch culture typically has traits that facilitate niksen, such as openness and freedom of movement and expression. And still, niksen can be very hard to do, no matter where you're from.

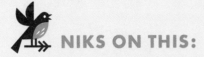

NIKS ON THIS:

• •

- Which lessons from the Dutch can you apply to
  your own life? Is it the concept of *gezelligheid*? Or
  maybe directness?

- If you could imagine a perfect place for niksen,
  what would it be?

- What do you think of the Netherlands as a
  country? Does my description make you want to
  move there?

CHAPTER 3

Why Is Niksen So Hard?

I'm sitting on the couch, trying to niks. I've been incredibly stressed out lately, and my heart is beating fast even though I'm desperately trying to relax. I should be calming down, but I'm not. Instead, I am noticing everything that needs to be done around the house, and I am acutely aware of the many deadlines pressuring me. I feel like I'm trying to catch a whole lot of eggs in a tiny basket and no matter how fast I run or how carefully I move, splashes of egg white and yolk are crashing onto the floor and furniture all around me. It is impossible to catch all these eggs.

I'm caught in a dilemma. On the one hand, I desperately need a break from the house, from the children, and from my work. From everything. But on the other hand, I'm unable to just let go. I wonder why that is. This should be easy, I think. After all, I'm not *doing* anything. I'm not running around cleaning and taking care of the house. I'm not working. The children are at school. This should be easy, but it's not.

When I sit down to take a little break, my thoughts begin to run wild in my head, chasing one another. Thinking about work becomes thinking about chores and that becomes thinking about my children. I worry. I wonder if I've done enough. And my laptop and mobile phone keep calling my name. Am I missing work opportunities? What if my friends are in trouble? What if I missed a Very Important Parenting Article that will tell me I am ruining my children's lives? To hell with niksen, I think, and I get up off the couch.

Sometimes busyness is the easy way out. It's easier to continue doing whatever you're doing, checking off items on your to-do list all day, than to stop, sit down, and do niks. In fact, in today's busy world, doing nothing can be the hardest thing to do.

When I look at the animal kingdom, I notice we are the only beings who never sit still. I wonder if all this is natural. Even great hunters like lions and fast runners like cheetahs take time to lounge about and do nothing. How did we lose the ability to sit still? And what price are we paying for this loss?

In the Spotlight

Timothy Wilson's "Shocking" Study

Niksen is uncomfortable. So uncomfortable that you might prefer to give yourself electric shocks than sit still for a while. That's exactly what a famous study by Timothy Wilson, a renowned psychologist at the University of Virginia, concluded.

"If thinking for pleasure is an engaging, enjoyable activity, participants should not feel the need to administer themselves unpleasant shocks," Wilson says. But somehow, they did just that.

Wilson and his colleagues hypothesized that what they called "thinking for pleasure" (and I call niksen) wouldn't be pleasant for participants. They wondered what would happen if they gave participants a choice between doing nothing and an unpleasant activity. So they devised a two-part study. In part one, participants rated the pleasantness of a series of stimuli, some of which were positive (like attractive photographs) and some negative (like a mild electric shock). In part two, participants were left alone for fifteen minutes and instructed to enjoy their thoughts.

(89)

They learned that the shock apparatus was still active and that they could receive shocks at the push of a button. The authors explained that their goal should be to enjoy their thoughts and that it was entirely up to them whether to press the shock button. What happened was that 67 percent of men and 25 percent of women gave themselves at least one shock during the thinking period.

This is remarkable given that people are usually pain avoidant. We instinctively try to minimize pain and maximize pleasure. And yet, we would rather shock ourselves than do nothing. The researchers concluded that thinking for pleasure, or niksen, is just no fun.

Where Does All the Busyness Come From?

Long ago, in ancient times, privileged groups in society began to flaunt their wealth in displays of conspicuous leisure. Engaging in activities that were obviously unproductive was a signal to the world around them to say, "Hey, look, I can afford not to work." This is known as *otium,* a Latin term with a variety of definitions that all imply some sort of leisure. The famous Roman scholar Cicero believed that a certain class in society should be able to spend their days in this kind of constant leisure.

Yet there has always been tension between the dream of leading a life of leisure and the desire to be productive. In medieval Europe, sloth was seen as a sin and work was viewed favorably. But working for many hours for solely financial reasons was seen as greed and therefore just as sinful as sloth. In the Bible, work was also presented as punishment.

As Irina Dumitrescu, a teacher of medieval literature

(90)

at the University of Bonn, says, "It's a question of balance. Leisure was certainly also viewed positively, and taking breaks was not seen as bad per se."

That said, people in medieval times rarely sat around and did nothing. "It's not that they were never relaxing," says Dumitrescu, "but they were always working. Work included not just their profession but also cooking, gardening, and praying." In fact, it was only after the industrial revolution that the difference between work and leisure became clear and, with time, that a whole industry devoted to helping us relax emerged.

Busy People, Everywhere

The truth is that we're busy and we're stressed. We feel overwhelmed by the business of our daily lives and this causes us to feel out of breath, rushed, and anxious. Desperate for a solution, we look for answers everywhere, even beyond the borders of our own country, hoping the next book or article will help us feel calmer and more able to live up to our expectations, obligations, and duties.

According to a Gallup poll in 2019, of 150,000 people surveyed around the world, Americans are particularly stressed out. The poll gathered data on both positive experiences (with questions like, Did you smile a lot yesterday? Were you treated with respect all day yesterday?) and negative experiences (Did you experience pain, sadness, worry, or anger yesterday?). Not only were Americans more stressed than people in other countries, they were also the most stressed they have been in a decade. The Gallup poll showed that being under fifty years old, having a low income, and not being a fan of President Trump were associated with mental health struggles. But Americans are not alone: globally, negative feelings were found to be at levels comparable to 2017, which was the most depressing year measured until now.

In an online article in *Psychology Today*, psychologist Jean M. Twenge explains that while people may not be admitting to depression, there is a clear increase in psychosomatic symptoms. "College students were 50% more likely to say they felt overwhelmed, and adults were more likely to say their sleep was restless, that they had poor appetite, and that everything was an effort—all classic psychosomatic symptoms of depression. But when people were asked directly if they 'felt depressed,' that didn't change much between the 1980s and the 2010s."

Twenge is best known for an article in *The Atlantic* in which she argued that smartphones are responsible for an epidemic of depression in teenagers. According to her, increased depression is related to the fact that our relationships and community ties are weaker, we have become more focused on tangible but material goals like money, and our expectations are ever growing. As you can imagine, in this context, it's unlikely people are doing a lot of niks.

The situation isn't much better in the UK. Yougov, a global opinion and data company, studied stress levels in that country and found that in 2017, 74 percent of British people were so stressed that they were unable to cope. Almost half the respondents stated that stress contributed to unhealthy eating habits, one-third admitted to increased alcohol consumption, and 16 percent said they were smoking more due to stress. Almost half of those surveyed felt depressed and two-thirds felt anxious. Worryingly, one-third of respondents admitted to suicidal thoughts. Financial problems, social pressure to succeed, and housing worries were cited as main causes of stress, along with deteriorating health conditions of loved ones. Another poll of two thousand people by the *Mirror* showed that half of British people feel "time-poor" and the majority are "too stressed out to have fun."

So, no wonder my article in the *New York Times* about doing nothing was met with such a wide and enthusiastic response. Inhabitants of most Western countries are hungry for a day off and a bit of rest. Many nations would do well to look at countries like the Netherlands that offer plenty of paid time off, a great social security network, and a wonderful work-life balance.

The Birth of a New Industry
In the nineteenth century, a new movement emerged in the US: New Thought. While it was initially viewed as no more than a short-term antidote to the rigid doctrines of Calvinism, this philosophy of optimism and positivity has blossomed into the huge wellness industry we know today

(93)

—complete with books, coaches, and products, including cosmetics—which was valued at 4.75 billion dollars in 2019. It is still very much alive and it's growing.

New Thought stands in stark contrast to Calvinism, which Barbara Ehrenreich aptly describes as "socially imposed depression" in her book *Smile or Die: How Positive Thinking Fooled America and the World.* Yet some Calvinistic tendencies remain mostly intact in New Thought, such as the constant self-examination and what Barbara Ehrenreich calls "judgmentalism." "The American alternative to Calvinism was not to be hedonism or even just an emphasis on emotional spontaneity. To the positive thinker, emotions remain suspect and one's inner life must be subjected to relentless monitoring," Ehrenreich says. Another similarity between positive thinking (and wellness in general) and Calvinism is the enormous emphasis that is placed on work. Though to New Thought the expectation is not that you work with your hands or on your job or professional life, it is that you work on yourself.

Around the time the New Thought movement appeared, psychologists expanded their study of what can go wrong within a human being's mind to begin examining what makes us happy, and this is what made us look at countries that scored highly on happiness studies, like Scandinavia or the Netherlands.

It can be argued that this isn't all as positive as it sounds, because with all this knowledge about happiness, people are increasingly feeling obliged and pressured to actually be happy. As Barbara Ehrenreich points out in *Smile or Die*, if there are people out there who "get it right," the advocates of positive psychology seem to be saying that we should be able to follow their lead.

The beginning of the wellness movement was not limited to the United States. Toward the end of the nineteenth century and into the twentieth century, Europe began to see a variety of movements, collectively known as Life Reform, appear that focused on physical fitness, a more "natural" way of life, sexual liberation, and a distrust of authority. During this time Germany gave birth to kindergartens, where children could play freely and learn social skills. Germans who emigrated to the US took this idea with them to their new home country, nowadays in the form of preschools.

It was also within this time frame that Maximilian Oscar Bircher Brenner tried to cure tuberculosis patients with a better diet — and ended up changing how the world eats breakfast by creating müsli. It is unclear whether his therapy was effective, but writer Thomas Mann visited Bircher Brenner's sanatorium and fled, calling it a "hygienic prison." A little earlier, Sebastian Kneipp had come up with a type of hydrotherapy and the beginning of naturopathy. And last but not least, Rudolf Steiner created Waldorf schools, though not without some serious controversy, especially because of their use of alternative medicines and belief in reincarnation.

The vestiges of these movements are evident today. Children are encouraged to play outside, and adults engage in organized sports. Organic food is considered preferable. And while these are positive developments, I don't mean to paint Europe as a paradise. The Old Continent has become obsessed with wellness. "Not the world needs to be improved but the self," said an article in the German paper *Der Tagesspiegel* critical of the reform movement.

Busyness as an Alternative Status Symbol

In 1899, the American economist and sociologist Thorstein Veblen published *The Theory of the Leisure Class,* which was met with wide acclaim. In line with Cicero's ideas on *otium,* he predicted that the wealthy classes would devote themselves wholly to what he called "conspicuous leisure." The prediction made sense at the time, but it didn't get even close to coming true.

Instead, alongside the expected conspicuous spending on luxury items such as clothes, cars, or wines, busyness has now become the ultimate status symbol.

In Veblen's time, work was seen as virtuous, but that virtue was unrelated to a person's value on the job market. "Whereas today, if you are busy all the time it means you are sought after," explains Silvia Bellezza, a researcher who studies alternative status symbols at Columbia Business School. Busyness as a status symbol is especially visible in the US, where the Protestant work ethic is strong and the belief that hard work will get you to the top prevails.

In the Netherlands there is even an expression to describe this: *druk druk, lekker belangrijk,* or "busy busy, so important!" It is sometimes shortened to DDLB, and some people, mostly upper class, use it in response to the question "How are you?" Though it is said in a tongue-in-cheek sort of way, it didn't come out of the blue. Being busy has become a status symbol, even in the otherwise equality-conscious Netherlands.

While many in Europe may relate to busyness as a status symbol, this doesn't seem to be the case in all cultures. In Bellezza's native Italy, for example, busyness is considered a burden. "If you were to get back from your summer holidays in September and say you'd been working, in Italy, people would think of you as a loser," she says.

Bellezza sees a drawback to this more leisurely approach to working life. "The whole country is paralyzed in the month of August because nobody does any work. And I think when people do work, they're not very productive." That's why she considers the Nordic countries and the Netherlands to have found the perfect balance. "There is respect for leisure time, so when people are on holidays they are actually on holidays and they travel. But when they work, their productivity is very high," she tells me. Personally, I can attest to this. When workers came in to redo my family's kitchen, they told us it would take them three days. They were done in two.

The Changing Nature of Work

(97)

Thanks to recent technological inventions and developments, we can now do more work more efficiently. Our expectations for ourselves (and others) have increased, as well as our options for how to spend our time. And

I'm not talking about just phones and computers. When my new kitchen was done, I found myself cooking much more because the food was ready in less time.

This happens at work as well. In this day and age "we are exposed to many things that just weren't an option before," says Tony Crabbe, a well-known business psychologist who works with large multinational companies such as IBM and Google. "Our expectations have as a result become stronger: we want to be better at doing more. We're supposed to be uber parents . . . as well as uber professionals." It seems all the technological advances that are supposed to make things easier for us actually end up putting more pressure on us.

This type of constant busyness and pressure is found especially among upper-middle-class professionals, says Crabbe, who noted that some of the most disengaged workers are some of the most highly educated, and the highest burnout rates are among the most educated, white-collar workers. "There is a feeling that overwhelm is taking over completely and the people who are writing about this and thinking about it are well-educated and well-off professionals," he said.

A contributing factor is what is known as the gig economy, an employment trend that relies on short-term workers and includes creatives, Uber drivers, and other small-business entrepreneurs, and increasingly also employees in more traditional industries. Short-term and project-based contracts are common but don't offer stability, and thus contribute to stress, busyness, and overwhelm. The idea that a person graduates, finds a job, and stays there until they retire has become a thing of the past. For more and more people, sitting back for a moment to relax may feel like a dangerous thing to do.

In his research, Paul Dolan found that working longer hours doesn't make us happier. Instead, there is an optimal number of working hours that is different for everyone, and working less than or more than that amount makes people unhappy.

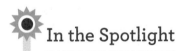 ## In the Spotlight

Niksen, Men, and Women

It turns out it is much easier for men to do nothing than it is for women.

Studies show that in heterosexual relationships, men don't just have more time than women, they are also much better at protecting the free time they have. And what's more, women protect their husbands' free time too, even at the expense of their own leisure, as Brigid Schulte discusses in *Overwhelmed: Work, Love, and Play When No One Has the Time.*

(99)

Statistics show that while men and women do approximately the same amount of work, men do more paid work while women do more unpaid work. This is the case all over the world, even in the most gender-equal countries, and progress in this respect seems to have flatlined. Even in Nordic countries, gender equality seems to be more a dream than a reality. We have come far, but not nearly far enough.

"I think we hold men and women's leisure time to different standards. We allow men to participate in daily relaxation, unwinding, and processing as their due for working," says Gemma Hartley, the journalist who popularized the term *emotional labor*.

Women, on the other hand, are allowed to niks but along more defined lines: "We generally don't mean zoning out, relaxing, or sitting down in your own house. We expect women to plan and work toward effortful self-care — a yoga class, a night out with the girls, a book club meeting — making women's leisure time exceptional rather than routine," says Hartley, admitting that she feels guilty when she reads a book on the couch while her husband does the dishes.

"There is no quiet moment, and if there is, we scramble to figure out what it is we're forgetting to do or we frantically fill that space with more." Doing nothing is practically unheard of among women. "It's a radical notion to say that we should do less, but ultimately one I think most women would benefit from embracing," she tells me in an email.

Still, men struggle with niksen too. Ludo Gabriele, a French writer living in the US with his wife, Diana, and their two children, fills me in: "As men, our sense of self and our social value are so attached to what we do, what we contribute, and what we provide that the absence of action can feel like a loss of self," he says. Gabriele is the man behind a blog called *Woke Daddy*, which aims to dismantle toxic masculinity.

And while men are stepping up at home and in their marriages, they're still acting "within restrictive gender norms. Those norms pressure us to exist in a narrow man-box that denies us a big portion of our humanity." These gender norms force men to close themselves off emotionally, which hinders their emotional development. "This leads to a myriad of harmful consequences such as anxiety, depression, and the inability to be in touch with ourselves and to form authentic relationships," he tells me via email.

These restrictive gender norms are a reality in the Netherlands too. "Traditional gender roles still persist in this country. Women do more unpaid care work, men bring home the bacon," says Suzan Steeman, an editor working for WomenInc., a network of women pushing for more gender equality. "We're progressive on the surface. But you need to look deeper," says Steeman. Her advice? "What is your ideal?" she asks me. In other words, you set your own terms. Think about what would be fair and equal for you and try to bring that into your own life.

Technology

One day, I set out to meet my Dutch teacher to see an exhibition she had organized, and I forgot to bring something of crucial importance: my phone. As a result, I couldn't find the place I was supposed to go to, and I couldn't let her know I wasn't going to make it. Not my proudest moment.

Tired and frustrated, I took the bus back home. It's such a little thing, a smartphone. But its absence had determined the course of my day, and it was a reminder of just how powerful but also how distracting technology is. I love having so much information at my fingertips. In fact, that trip reminded me of how in the past, I often had to just deal with not knowing something. Now, thanks to having our devices constantly on hand, we can know pretty much everything, anywhere and anytime.

There is so much we can know that we are often distracted. Doreen Dodgen-Magee researches how technology affects both our interpersonal connections and our ability to be idle. She found that many people self-soothe with screens and devices, and she began to wonder how that was impacting people's ability to have a real, strong, cohesive sense of self. "Instead of looking inside of ourselves and being able to soothe ourselves and know how to feel about ourselves, we are now looking outside of ourselves and to our devices. We have an external locus of control instead of an internal locus of control," she says, referring to the principle in psychology that describes the degree to which people believe they have control over their lives. The result of the external locus is that we constantly want to engage with our devices "and the cycle just starts feeding itself," Dodgen-Magee says. We want to feel better, and we believe that our devices will give us that feeling.

According to Chris Bailey, we'd all do much better resisting the urge to grab our devices and scroll away, because all that switching, browsing, and scrolling is not just unproductive but also bad for our attention span. So not only have we become dependent on our phones for self-soothing, but we also are more scattered, more distracted, and more stressed out. And it's only a few moments before we reach for our phones . . . a vicious cycle.

Technology also blurs the lines between our private lives and our work. We can check our email at midnight, make a Skype call before the sun is up to speak to a client in a different time zone, or do research all day and night on the internet. With these options available, our ideas about work have changed too: employers expect employees to be available at all times while employees can never really turn work off.

Technology also blurs the lines between work and leisure because so much of what we do for leisure is a lot like what we do at work. When I admit to psychologist Sandi Mann that I spent a lot of time browsing Facebook and calling it research, she admits to the same and adds an interesting point: "Exactly. I'm always scrolling Facebook and calling it research. But interestingly, when

(103)

you're scrolling, you're performing a very similar activity, the same activity you do when you're genuinely doing research."

Changing Expectations

When we think of busyness, we usually think of work. But the overwhelm spills over into other areas of our lives too. For example, not only are we spending more time at work, parents are also spending more and more time with their children. And this is true for both moms and dads. Men have become increasingly involved husbands and fathers and also perform more chores than their own fathers did, so they spend much more time being busy with the home. That said, women still do the majority of housework and childrearing.

While spending more time with the children and the family appears to be a positive development, for many it can actually create increased levels of stress and busyness. This is especially true in homes where the parents (or one of the parents) are employed in what the *New York Times* calls "greedy work," or work that requires extraordinary commitment. Think very long hours and the expectation that you work as though you have zero social or personal life. Professionals in the worlds of finance, law, and consulting are especially at risk of falling prey to greedy work, and this can create stress and busyness for both parents and children.

But it's not just professional expectations; add to this the fact that social expectations of parents have also risen, and you have a recipe for disaster. These days, many parents feel it's not enough to just feed their children on time. They feel pressured to serve organic, GMO-free, and homemade food that takes hours to prepare. And instead of simply raising and loving children the best way they can, there is a pressure to be up-to-date on the countless parenting books and trends. For many parents, figuring out what their parenting philosophy is and putting that into practice is a task that is given tremendous focus and attention.

Wired for Busyness?

There might be a reason we'd rather give ourselves electric shocks than be idle, and it's not culture. It's nature. We might, in fact, be hardwired for busyness. As Sandi Mann tells me: "There's an evolutionary benefit to us being busy, to being active. We're not designed to be sitting there. We're designed to be active and to be constantly searching our environment, trying to improve things."

In ancient times, people just sitting around could be eaten by a saber-toothed tiger or some other now long-extinct animal. And because in the past resources were scarce, early humans constantly had to search for, worry about, and collect those resources. Someone who is being idle isn't doing any of these things.

"They're not searching for food and they're not on the lookout for danger either," observes Sandi Mann of idle people. "Nowadays, intellectual skills are valued. But in the past, those weren't appreciated; it was what you could do with your hands, what you could grow in the field, what you could catch. Those were the skills that were praised. Sitting and thinking aren't skills that we're designed to value."

Only much later, after the dawn of agriculture, could a certain class of people devote their days to Thinking Big Thoughts and not worrying about food, while other people were busy doing that for them.

Dopamine Hit

One of the reasons we love being busy is the way it makes us feel. "We probably get a dopamine hit, the feel-good chemical, from being active. We certainly get dopamine hits from novelty. And to experience those new things we need to stay active," explains Sandi Mann.

Being busy makes us feel productive and like we have our lives under control. There is a reason why to-do lists and bullet journals are so popular: the sense of satisfaction that can be found when we divide the day into small, manageable chunks. When we view the day in this simple, linear way and assign ourselves clear tasks — first work, then laundry, then dinner — and attend to these tasks one by one, ticking them off as we complete them, we feel productive and satisfied.

Humans like to set goals for themselves, however small

(although my mountain of laundry is anything but small), and then work toward accomplishing them and toward that satisfied, productive feeling. But when our tasks become too many, that's when we begin to feel busy.

One of the evolutionary reasons why we stay busy is of a more indirect nature and has to do with the deeply embedded human need for connection and belonging. Despite the fact that many of us — myself included — may be introverted or even people avoidant, in general we are a highly social species. According to renowned psychologist Matthew Lieberman, in his book *Social: Why Our Brains Are Wired to Connect,* we devote time and attention to observing how people around us behave, speak, think, and feel. He even considers our social abilities something of a superpower. Sometimes, however, this superpower works against us.

For instance, when we see others constantly very busy, we feel the pressure to be the same. If we don't join in, the price — socially speaking — is potentially high. But if everyone around us is always focused on some task, we begin to feel weird if we don't follow suit. We begin to wonder what's wrong with us. In fact, brain scans have shown that when respondents are asked to recall recent rejections, the parts of the brain that light up are associated with physical pain. Not fitting in literally hurts. And there are further risks associated with feelings of rejection or isolation, such as depression and decreased mental and physical health outcomes

While it is absolutely possible to resist the peer pressure of busyness when you live in a society with a strong work ethic, it's very, very hard.

Or Are We Wired for Niksen Too?

As important as it was to collect food for the tribe, be on the lookout for saber-toothed tigers, and make tools and clothing for the family, all of that requires a lot of energy. And even though we are wired to be busy, we are also wired to save energy. In fact, looking at how our eating patterns have developed over the centuries, it can safely be concluded that we are a fabulously lazy species.

Hunting a mammoth may seem like a great idea. It would mean a lot of food for a whole tribe, but it would require hours of running after a huge animal and involve a high chance of getting killed. It would also require extreme energy from both you and your fellow hunters. Too much effort really, which is why prehistoric hunter-gatherer humans typically settled on a few hare traps and a handful of berries instead.

"People are more attracted to doing nothing. If they have the opportunity to take the escalator or to take the stairs, most of them will take the escalator. Because it will save energy, they won't have to do anything," explains Matthieu Boisgontier, the French researcher on inactivity. We bring this attitude to most of what we do. We work toward becoming increasingly efficient so as to ensure our survival at minimum effort. Long ago, the more efficient we became, the easier it was to find food and the more time we had to recharge the energy we expended during our activities. Now we've actually become so efficient at saving energy that we have created all sorts of problems.

"We're not really trying to be active. We're just trying to be as inactive as we can, physically speaking. And now that's a problem, because we don't have to run after our food anymore," he says. Boisgontier's theory is that we're attracted to what he calls "task minimization" because we hate to waste energy. We're wired for busyness. But we're wired for niksen too.

Guilty Pleasure

When I first started researching niksen, I thought that only people in Western cultures might feel guilty for not working and that other parts of the world were more likely to enjoy time off work with more abandon. But then I talked to intercultural researcher Eleonore Breukel and that view quickly came apart.

When we think of time off, we may not always think of doing nothing. We may instead think of spending time with our families, going out with friends, or performing religious duties. "I think that in other cultures this is also true and maybe more so than in the West, but being with extended family is certainly not doing nothing. It is doing something, and it can take quite some energy. Even if we see it as free time . . . No, it's not free time," she tells me. "In many non-Western cultures, people are expected to participate in all sorts of duties and tasks, be it religious

(109)

duties, for instance, or maybe family obligations. I don't think this sounds so relaxing, although we may consider it time off."

Many feelings come up around doing nothing and taking time off. The most profound of these feelings, experienced by people all over the world, is guilt. In the West, guilt brings many mixed messages and opposing feelings: we feel guilty for not working but we may also feel guilty for working too much. Sometimes we even end up feeling guilty for feeling guilty, which is particularly challenging to deal with.

"We feel guilty when we're not with our kids and when we're not working. That's a double whammy of guilt if you're taking some time off just for yourself. There is definitely the feeling that we should be doing stuff," says Sandi Mann, the British psychologist and expert on boredom.

Silvia Bellezza, an Italian researcher who has been living in the US for the last twelve years, told me, "I grew up in a system that slows down a lot in the summer and around Christmastime. I cannot work 365 days a year. My brain doesn't work on Christmas Day. So, I try to unplug. I try to emulate the system of the Scandinavian countries. When I have time off, I really disconnect. It's not easy to do.

"I really like my work here, but the work mentality in this country definitely changes you a lot," she says, admitting that she used to be reluctant to use an out-of-

office assistant because she didn't want people to know she was on holiday. When I ask her whether she feels guilty in both Italy and the US, she says, "I definitely do feel guilty in Italy when I work on a Sunday instead of being with my parents."

While guilt is an unpleasant emotion, it is somehow refreshing to know that we're not the only ones experiencing it. Guilt, it seems, is an emotion that connects us all.

What Does Busyness Do to Us?

Complaining about our stressful lives is a daily occurrence; I am sure you've heard people do it. You may have even done it yourself. We throw the word *stress* around quite a bit, but do we really know what it means? Let's take a closer look. Just a little caveat before I continue: I am not a doctor, just a writer who has researched stress and its negative effects on the human body and mind and interviewed various experts on the topic.

We feel stressed out when we're faced with a situation that would require us to change or adjust our behavior or circumstances. Stress is actually an important reaction to any situation that needs our attention. But too much stress, and we're in trouble.

When I ask Carolien Hamming what stress is, she tells me it is "your body's adaptive reaction. We experience stress not just at work, but also when we engage in sports because we need energy and stress gives us that energy." Stress is a bodily reaction that can occur with any

(111)

type of activity. "You can feel stress any time you're active." There's a positive correlation between the level of stress and the level of activity: "The more active we are, the more stress we feel," explains Hamming.

Generally speaking, stress is a positive and important reaction. It's like pain in that it tells us when something is wrong and that we have to do something about that. Stress is nature's way of telling us that we need time to unwind. But just like the frog that doesn't feel the temperature of the water rising and ends up slowly being boiled to death, we often don't notice how stressed we are until it's too late.

"When you then sit down and do niks, you notice how stressed your body is. You notice you can't calm down. You can't tell yourself 'now I want to calm down'; it doesn't work that way," Carolien Hamming says. Our bodies adapt to elevated stress levels and begin to consider that level the new normal. "Your body adapts, your brain adapts," according to Hamming. She compares stress to a wave with peaks of heightened activity and valleys of calm downtime. But when we're chronically stressed, "the peaks become bigger and last longer and we can't go back down into downtime," she explains.

"Too much stress causes the body to go into fight-or-flight mode. When this happens, our nervous system jumps into overdrive, which can cause symptoms of anxiety to arise, as well as insomnia and irritability," reports Juli Fraga, a psychologist and writer based in San Francisco who specializes in emotional well-being, mental health, and parenthood.

Chronic stress, says Fraga, can "also dampen one's immune system, making people more prone to colds and flus. Stress also causes bodily tension, which can lead to muscular aches and pains." And once your stress response system has been activated, it generally takes a while for it to calm down. Stress is a full-body response, requiring the cooperation of various systems. Shutting down that response requires all those systems to agree to let go.

Stress can even rewire our brains to think this is a normal state of being, thanks to what is known as neuroplasticity. Neuroplasticity, or brain plasticity, is the ability of the brain to change continuously throughout an individual's life. "It's not just behavioral that we have a hard time being still and being quiet. It's also that we have actually rewired our brains so that the parts of the brain related to stillness and emotional regulation have been pruned," says Doreen Dodgen-Magee.

For most of us, stress causes anxiety. "Stress can activate our 'inner critics,' that internal voice that tells us we aren't good enough, smart enough, or capable of handling the demands of life," says Fraga. And this voice increases stress levels because it makes us want to do more, not less, so that we don't feel so inadequate. "As a result, not only is there more stress but also feelings of irritability and anxiety arise."

When we become too anxious or stressed out, we lose focus, are unable to work, and struggle with even the simplest, most basic everyday tasks. This spirals into a vicious cycle, as we are unable to do our work and fall behind, which leads to more anxiety and more stress. Stress is the path to the dark side. Stress leads to worry. Worry leads to anxiety. Anxiety leads to suffering. Another vicious circle. (Feel free to read this in your best Yoda voice.)

In his book *Busy: How to Thrive in a World of Too Much,* Tony Crabbe focuses on the effect busyness has on our ability to retain focused attention. "For me, the opposite of busyness isn't relaxation on the beach, it's the ability to focus on what matters more despite this crazy tsunami of other people or problems," he says. He suggests that stress doesn't just affect companies and organizations where too much stress, and a decreased focus level, might lead to slower progress, but also increasingly affects family dynamics.

The Bright Side of Busyness

All this busyness has a bright side too. "There are reasons we work so much. Part of it is has to do with the pressures of careers and markets, but the other side of the story is that there are a lot of fun things to do. For most people, work is more interesting than it was a hundred years ago," says Ruut Veenhoven.

Unfortunately, though, while work for many may have

become more interesting, intellectually challenging, and creative, it has also led to the emergence of a new kind of stress: FOMO, or the fear of missing out. There are so many fun things to do that we become anxious about our choices. Choosing one activity or job or project means saying no to another, and many of us live with the constant feeling that there is something better for us right around the corner, something we can't see or just said no to. We work a little harder, trying to fit more into our day. And this isn't true for just our professional lives; socially we can have the same constant anxiety and resulting busyness.

"I think we're afraid that if we don't fill up every moment, we're not using our time fully and productively. So, whenever we have a little time we get onto the internet and all these devices and swipe and scroll away. We're not allowing ourselves any downtime for our minds to just be free and still," explains Sandi Mann.

Always being busy has become a familiar feeling: we are used to it, know it well, and everyone around us knows what it's like to feel busy too. As a result, we've created a society that thinks busyness is normal or even desirable. It actually crept up on us, but now it's all we know. "Humans will always choose the familiar over the unknown. We have taught ourselves to believe that the best way to be is to be productive. We now easily choose the familiar path of busyness rather than letting ourselves sit in the discomfort of having nothing to do," says Doreen Dodgen-Magee.

Wrapping It Up

In this chapter we went through the many reasons why we are so busy and had a look at how modern technology sometimes exacerbates the feeling of busyness by keeping us distracted and connected at all times. We saw how the way we work makes it very hard for us to do nothing because the lines between our private and working lives have become blurred. All these factors make niksen difficult, but not impossible. Because while you learned that we might actually be hardwired for busyness, you also saw that we're a fabulously lazy species. So not all hope is lost —one day niksen might come naturally after all.

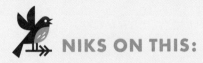

NIKS ON THIS:

....

- When do you feel stressed out?

- How does your relationship with technology contribute to this?

- And how does it affect you and the people around you?

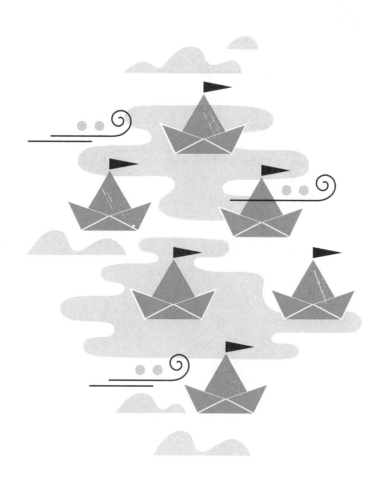

Niksen Is Good for You. Yes, It Is.

Once again, I'm on my couch. This time I'm not working or thinking, or even reading. I'm niksening, and it is delicious. I feel relaxed, and just sitting here feels good. Every now and then I feel the urge to get up and take care of the laundry, but I ignore it because, finally, I'm in the niksen zone.

For a few glorious moments there is nothing demanding my attention. I feel the stress seeping out of me. I'm relaxed but alert, ready to take on the day. And after a while, I notice something happening. Ideas begin to form and float around in my head. They bump into one another and become new ideas, each one more original than the one preceding it.

Moments like this rarely last long. Soon, the whirlwind of chores and duties will overtake me again, as it always does. But this moment right here? It's great, I think to myself. I could use more of this.

When I get up to work a little later, the words flow

easily, and I even find myself breezing through my most hated chores without a fuss. I feel like it's easier to make decisions, and I'm happier, more at ease, with the ones I've made. I feel charged with a sort of superpower that makes almost everything possible.

My day is not really less busy than usual, my obligations aren't in any way fewer. I still have all my work and the children and the house, day in and day out. But somehow, after this brief but powerful moment of respite, I feel better equipped to deal with all that is expected of me. Even though there are duties jumping at me like they always are, I handle them like a boss. And I even feel creative, playful, and productive. So the question is, how does this flow state relate to niksen?

Your Brain and Body on Niksen

"The conventional way to find out how the brain works is to ask it to do something. You create a task," Marcus Raichle, an American neurologist and professor at the Washington University School of Medicine, tells me.

For a long time, the dominant belief was that when we're not doing anything, our brains aren't either. But this is not what Raichle found when he put people in an fMRI scanner, which measures brain activity by detecting changes associated with blood flow to certain areas of the brain. When an area in the brain is in use, there is an increase of blood flow to that region.

"I was surprised to find that when you engage in a task, some areas of the brain actually decrease in activity," he tells me over the phone. By contrast, when participants laid still and were not engaged in a specific task, something amazing happened. A special network that included all the major connections in the brain lit up.

Raichle now calls this the default mode network. "Your brain is always active, always on," he says, even when you're not doing anything. Raichle had set out to map the brain when people were not doing anything in particular, and instead of less activity, he saw areas with increased activity. What's more, this special network always involved the same areas of the brain.

In other words, niksen is our default state, from which we "awaken" only when motivated by some inner drive, anxiety, or external stimuli. For me, it's the vision of a clean room (even if said room will remain clean for a total of only five minutes, and that's if I'm lucky). And when we set about doing a task, we engage certain parts of the brain and shut down others.

"The brain acts in a very coordinated way when you're lying in the scanner. When you're doing nothing, your brain is doing a whole lot," he continues. As he speaks, I find myself becoming more and more fascinated. Our brains have a whole network of neural connections devoted to . . . doing nothing? Wait, what?

This is not to imply that when we're focused on a task our neural pathways aren't at work. It makes sense that the brain directs energy and resources to the parts required for the task at hand, but this isn't at the expense of any other vital activities. Raichle, who plays the oboe in his free time, compares the parts of the brain to the members of an orchestra.

"There are seventy-five people on the stage, and the music is a combination of the way they come together. Each instrument and musician is part of a larger picture," he tells me. Sometimes all the instruments play together, and sometimes the piano or the violin stands out. Soloists and the ensemble work together to create a harmonious sound, and all are necessary for the whole to come together and function.

Raichle's discovery has been met with some skepticism, mostly because we don't know exactly what the brain does in default mode. The theory that this mode is responsible for creativity and mind wandering could be a premature conclusion. Yet Raichle is certainly on to something, and his discovery of the default mode network has changed the way we talk about the brain. We no longer think in terms of centers (for example, a center for language and a center for creative thought and a center for calculating) but now speak about large-scale brain networks — for example, the default mode network, the dorsal and ventral attention networks (which are responsible for our voluntary and involuntary reactions to new events), the salience network (which measures how important external and internal events are to us), the fronto-parietal network (which modulates cognitive function), and the lateral visual network (which has to do with emotions). These are just a few of the largest brain networks, and many others have been found since.

Raichle believes the default mode is an essential mode for the brain to be in. "It's important for this system to be active. It's amazing, all the things that are going on in your brain, talking quietly to itself, when there is no task at hand."

When I ask him what the brain is doing when it's not doing anything, he pauses and replies, "Everything."

Redefining Productivity

"I bet you've spent a hundred hours on an article and it didn't come out very well. And then you spent twelve hours on another article and it was a big hit," Robert Pozen, a professor of management at MIT and the author of *Extreme Productivity: Boost Your Results, Reduce Your Hours,* teases me. I nod because he is absolutely right. I have written articles and blog posts that took almost no time yet were very well read and highly appreciated. And I have also spent countless hours on a story only to have it flop.

(123)

"So, when were you more productive?" he asks me, and then answers the question himself:

"I'd say you were more productive during the twelve hours because you focused, you figured out what the audience wanted, you got your priorities right, you communicated well." Yet boasting that I spent a hundred hours on an article sounds much more impressive.

To Pozen, the hours we spend on something is not what we should be proud of. At work and in life, we live by the mantra that the more hours we spend on something, the better it must be. The more time we spend at the office, we think, the harder we work. We measure value in the number of hours spent. And we shouldn't.

"You see it all the time. Someone will believe, *I'm a great employee because I am at work every night 'til 10 p.m.* The question is, is that really true?" says Pozen. "If you're reading about productivity, you should hopefully get this time back and be able to work and live smarter. And not all advice lives up to that."

What Chris Bailey calls mind-wandering and I call niksen is great advice for anyone looking to be more productive. "Because we don't have to force ourselves to focus on anything, we replenish our supply of energy when our mind wanders. And so we get that time back and then some," he says.

In our modern working culture, we mistake working long hours for getting things done. We also focus on things that can be visibly measured rather than on what actually matters.

"We feel more productive on a day spent answering every single email in our inbox than a day spent mentoring two new employees who joined our team. Yet if you add up all the cascading effects of mentoring those two employees," says Bailey, "the outcome might be huge. Maybe they stay on at the company. Maybe they are happier, they are better motivated. Maybe they help others more," Bailey muses. But the results of this mentoring can be seen only in the future and lack a sense of urgency, so most will feel more productive emptying the inbox.

"You should not be focusing on how many hours you work, but on that you get a lot accomplished," agrees Robert Pozen of MIT.

Sometimes doing nothing will be just what you need to become a more productive human being. Maybe you just need to redefine productivity so that you can feel productive lying on the couch, or taking care of your family, or going to a museum, or doing something else that doesn't have an immediate purpose or a measurable outcome.

 ## In the Spotlight

Procrastination

Procrastination can look a lot like niksen. But "there's a fine line between 'doing nothing' to promote wellness and decrease stress, and procrastination," says Juli Fraga. The difference is in our reasons for doing nothing. "When we're enjoying downtime, we aren't avoiding something," she says. But when we procrastinate, we are avoiding a particular activity "because we want to stave off the feeling that doing it triggers."

(125)

Some people like to pretend they're not really procrastinating but working, and they start to organize their bookshelves by color, go through old emails, or clean the house. This can be an insidious way of procrastinating because it looks so much like work.

"If you're in bed watching a movie, you know you're procrastinating. But if you're vacuuming, if you're going through your files, getting them organized, going through old emails, alphabetizing your bookshelves, that feels like 'oh, I'm being productive.' So you're not feeling the weight of procrastination as deeply," explains author Gretchen Rubin.

Niksen can help with procrastination by giving us a very clear time and place for not doing anything, and then, with renewed energy, we might feel more content to get back to work and finish what we've started (or start what we need to finish).

For a while, I thought all procrastinators were the same, but this couldn't be further from the truth. There can be many situations that cause us to procrastinate, and there are three types of procrastinators, according to Rubin:

1. The Anxious Procrastinator
"People feel anxious about a task, so they don't want to start. Your anxiety builds as you procrastinate and then probably your deadline is looming," says Gretchen Rubin, and I nod because this sounds way too familiar. "Finally, your fear of missing the deadline overwhelms

your anxiety and so you start, but it's already too late. Now you're anxious, you have limited the amount of time you have to make your deadline, and you may not be doing your best work."

2. The Disgusted Procrastinator
The disgusted procrastinator may not even have a deadline. He or she just really has absolutely no desire to do the task that needs to be done. "It's not anxiety, it's just distaste. It's like, 'ugh,'" Rubin tells me. I immediately think of how I feel about cleaning.

3. The Manipulative Procrastinator
Some people procrastinate because they hope that someone will come in and rescue them from their obligations somehow. "They say, 'Hey, if I don't take out the trash, maybe you'll come home and you'll be so disgusted by the trash that you'll just do it,'" Rubin says.

Niksen and Creativity: Why Do the Best Ideas Happen in the Shower?

"I took people off the street and took them to a sound-proof room, and I asked them to leave their phones behind. And I said we want to see how you'll feel," says psychologist Sandi Mann. At first, people were very uncomfortable, but after a while, they eased into being there with nothing to do, and they came out feeling calmer and more relaxed. This experiment was specifically aimed at discovering whether doing nothing would make people more creative. And it did.

"I've given people creativity tests, and the people who were bored were more creative than the people who weren't," Mann explains. The creativity tests involved providing as many answers as possible to a series of word problems and the results were clear: boredom literally makes us more creative, better at problem solving, better at coming up with creative ideas. But being bored wasn't defined as sitting in front of a computer aimlessly scrolling or tweeting your way through the day. In the experiment it was important that the mind was given space to daydream and wander free from distractions. I feel this experiment was therefore not about boredom at all. It was a study of niksen.

"We need you to be really lazy and literally be doing nothing. Let your mind be totally bored and let it search for its own stimulation," Sandi Mann says. Maybe this is why the line between doing nothing and doing creative work can sometimes become so blurry.

Chris Bailey is an avid knitter and tells me that this helps him relax and let his mind wander. "Because of this wandering, our minds go off into places where we can connect ideas that we had in the past to problems that we're facing in the present, to decide how we're going to act on that problem in the future," he explains, telling me how new creative solutions come into being.

"Mind wandering connects the constellation of ideas

that are swirling around in our minds to become something new that we would not arrive at otherwise. That we would never arrive at if we were devoting our full attention to it," says Bailey.

That's why when we're taking a shower, or sitting on the couch, or knitting, or niksening around, ideas come together as if by magic. This quiet, seemingly passive work is less visible and less impressive than the more obvious eureka moments, but it's just as important.

I look at my own work and wonder, Was it the reading and constantly keeping my eyes open, the listening to what people are saying both online and offline that gave me the idea for an article? Or was it the quiet time I spent in between one project and the next that made the difference? In the first you would see me hard at work. But I know now the incubation period (niksen) is just as important.

 In the Spotlight

. . . .

Monty Python's John Cleese on Creativity

In a talk called "How to Be Creative," John Cleese of Monty Python says that people can get into one of two moods, or as he calls them, modes: closed and open. The closed mode is how we feel when we work. "It's a mode in which we're probably a little impatient, if only with ourselves. It has a little tension in it, and not

(129)

much humor. We're very purposeful, and it's a mode in which we can get very stressed and even a bit manic," he explains.

This is exactly how it feels to be on a deadline or to work toward something with purpose. It's effective and helps us get the work done but it's not very creative.

The open mode, by contrast, is a "relaxed . . . expansive . . . less purposeful mode . . . in which we're probably more contemplative, more inclined to humor (which always accompanies a wider perspective) and, consequently, more playful. It's a mood in which curiosity for its own sake can operate because we're not under pressure to get a specific thing done quickly. We can play, and that is what allows our natural creativity to surface."

His description of the open mode sounds to me exactly like niksen. The lack of distractions and sensory cues leaves people's minds looking for their own entertainment and coming up with more creative, inventive ideas. Though the seeds of these ideas were already there, the quiet and the niksen are what actually make creativity shine.

SPACE TO YOURSELF

According to Cleese, to be creative, "you have to create some space for yourself away from those demands. And that means sealing yourself off," he says.

The concept of space is, of course, fluid. It could mean an actual space like a writing desk in a separate room. And then there is also the mental space, which also needs to be sealed off from distractions.

TIME
Cleese says that not only do we need space to do creative work, we also need a certain yet definite amount of time to sit still.

"It's only by having a specific moment when your space starts and an equally specific moment when your space stops that you can seal yourself off from the everyday closed mode in which we all habitually operate," Cleese says.

Paradoxically, for creativity to be boundless, it needs to have boundaries.

We don't really need a whole morning or half a day to be creative. It doesn't have to be every day either. "It's far better to do an hour-and-a-half now and then an hour-and-a-half next Thursday and maybe an hour-and-a-half the week after that than to fix one four-and-a-half-hour session now," says Cleese.

And so it is for niksen too — it's good to schedule a little time for it. And a little is better than none at all.

MORE TIME
I thought we discussed time, I hear you say. But this is a different kind of time: the time required to sit with an idea for a while even if it's uncomfortable. "If we have a problem and we need to solve it, then until we do, we feel inside us a kind of internal agitation, a tension, or

(131)

an uncertainty that makes us just plain uncomfortable. And we want to get rid of that discomfort. So, in order to do so, we make a decision. Not because we're sure it's the best decision, but because making it will make us feel better," says Cleese.

The difference between creative and uncreative people is that "most creative people have learned to tolerate that discomfort for much longer. And so, just because they put in more pondering time, their solutions are more creative."

It's the same with niksen. It can feel quite unpleasant at times, which is why we quickly distract ourselves with our phones and screens. Learn to sit with that discomfort for a while and you will be surprised by the benefits niksen has to offer — and the creativity that springs from it.

Better Decision Makers Thanks to Niksen

I don't consider myself to be an intuitive person. I like going over a problem, viewing it from different perspectives, and choosing the option that seems most logical to me. When I rely on logical thinking to make decisions, I feel better than when I rely on my gut feeling. I once even wrote an article about this in which I argued that we should always choose logic over intuition. In his book *Thinking, Fast and Slow,* Nobel Prize winner Daniel Kahneman makes a passionate argument against intuition, calling it a "heuristic," or a shortcut, that saves us time but can lead to inaccurate decisions.

I talked to Dutch psychologist, professor, and happiness researcher Ap Dijksterhuis. He didn't exactly make me change my mind on the superiority of logic, but helped me appreciate the value of intuition just a little bit more. In five different experiments, he found that when people had to decide on highly complex matters, such as buying an apartment or choosing a roommate, their intuitive choices were much more accurate and they were more satisfied with their decisions.

In all the experiments, participants were divided into three groups: The first was told to make the decision immediately after being shown all the options. The second group had three minutes to choose and was encouraged to consciously consider the pros and cons of each decision. The third group was distracted with a task that had nothing to do with housing and then told to decide. In all five experiments, the group that was distracted with another task made the most accurate decisions. (Accuracy was measured by how well respondents were able to recognize the positive and negative aspects of every option.)

So while logic and conscious thought can be useful when making important life decisions, especially ones that don't include too many variables, this way of thinking has its limits.

"Intuition is so much more useful. In fact, if you don't have intuition and you have to force yourself to make a decision, the outcome is actually worse," Dijksterhuis tells me. But there is a catch to the method. To make accurate decisions using intuition, participants had to spend time doing nothing or being distracted by some other activity that had nothing to do with the decision. So next time you are faced with an important decision, just get onto your couch and niks around for a while.

Dijksterhuis tells me that when we use logic, our brains work in a linear manner, solving one issue after the other like in a math equation. Complex decisions, however, require us to solve several problems at the same time. "With conscious decisions, you think about the one or two most important things. With unconscious decisions, you think about so much more. And it helps when you're not focused," he explains.

So as faulty as our intuition may be, it can also lead us to the right choice. In *Thinking, Fast and Slow,* Daniel Kahneman discusses a study he conducted with Gary Klein, in which firefighters were able to successfully predict where a fire would cause the floor to collapse mere moments before it happened. The firemen felt the heat coming and knew when and how to withdraw based on experience and intuition. However, they proved less successful when faced with circumstances they had less experience with.

(134)

When we're short on time and don't have all the information we need, we can trust our instincts because that's exactly what they are for. Decisions made this way may not be optimal but are probably better than flipping a coin. (That said, when people flipped a coin to answer the question of whether they should change jobs, they were usually happier when they did, regardless of what the coin said. Go figure.)

Our intuition works well when we have expertise in a certain area and in "kind learning environments," or learning situations that provide immediate feedback so we can transform experiences and their consequences into gut feelings. For example, if your intuition tells you to use a certain spice in your cooking, the effect will be sensed immediately (when you taste the sauce and either smile or grimace) or when you serve the food. Next time you prepare dinner, you might reach for that spice again, or choose something else because that first intuition proved wrong.

Wrapping It Up

Niksen isn't a luxury; it's a necessity. Our bodies need it, and our brains need it too in order to do their work well. After a niksen break, we're not just better rested, we also have more clarity and are better equipped to face our day-to-day challenges. And in this lies the real power of niksen.

In this chapter, you learned how niksen can be good for your mental health by giving your body and mind a chance to rest. We also saw that it has positive effects on our creativity, as it allows ideas and solutions to bounce around and bump into one another, creating new connections. And niksen makes us more productive and better decision makers too because taking breaks from work makes us perform better and more efficiently. I'd like to argue, though, that we need to allow ourselves to take breaks just because, and not just so we can be efficient, creative, and productive. But a question still remains: How?

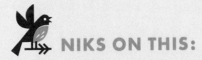

NIKS ON THIS:

. . . .

- How does doing nothing affect your productivity, creativity, and decision-making process?

- When was the last time you had a creative idea or solved a complex problem? And did it happen after a period of niksening?

- Can you think of other ways niksen is good for you?

Niksen Is Good for You. Yes, It Is.

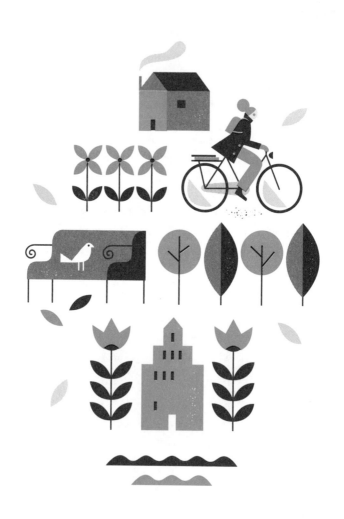

CHAPTER 5

Niksening Up Your Life

I talk about niksening on my couch a lot. But I must admit I could do with a little bit more of it. How can I become better at it? How can I niks up my life at work, at home, and out in public? Like most modern humans, I'm busy. Even though at times my life may look pretty leisurely, I *feel* busy most of the time. And that busyness is not doing me any good.

But niksen is hard! How can I make sure that I get enough niksen time on top of all my other duties and responsibilities? How can I niksen when I need to get my work done, take care of the children, and keep my house clean? And, most importantly, how can I enjoy my time on the couch instead of thinking about everything that I need to do?

Work, home, and the public space are the three most important areas of our lives. If we could introduce at least some niksen into all these spaces, that would be a huge step toward a calmer, more relaxed life. I notice that when I make time for niksen, or at least find some niksen pockets throughout the day, I become more relaxed. Those niksening moments seep into the rest of my life, making my day feel slower but so much more effective. I see how bringing niksen into one area affects the others in positive ways.

And, to my big surprise, I found out that niksen is not something that you can do only at home. On the contrary, the great thing about it is that you can niks anywhere, no matter who you are or what you have with you.

Here's how.

Niksen at Work

Why postpone your niksen time until you get back home when you can do it at work? In fact, you need breaks and time to relax in the office too. This won't be good just for you but for your employer as well. Here's how to bring niksen to your job.

Make Time to Do Nothing, and Do It on Purpose
Whether at work or at home, figure out when you're at your most productive and creative, then notice when your mind starts to shut off or when you start performing tasks on autopilot. That's when you should go for a walk or take a break. This, according to productivity expert Chris Bai-

ley, won't just help you relax and make you more productive, it might also neutralize some of that niksen-related guilt. If you want to do nothing, the first order of business is to stop working. This is commonly referred to as "taking a break," and in our busy culture, it seems to be a rare habit. We see people eating lunch at their desks (or, as Li Bruno put it, "al desko") trying to be more productive, but ironically, they're not. Instead, they are heading straight to burnout town.

Robert Pozen of MIT tells me that "after sixty to ninety minutes, people start to lose attention and are less focused" and ideally this is when they should take a break. What's more, there are several types of breaks. "There's a break at the ground level, so taking short breaks throughout the day. And then there is the level above that, which is taking longer breaks from work. In terms of these longer breaks from work, we deserve two or three of those a year," says Chris Bailey, who then candidly admits to not taking as many vacation days as he should.

Still, he tries to take a few days off at a time, "just to relax, and process information and read."

Resist the Culture of Busyness

If you're doing nothing, own it. When someone asks you what you're doing during your niksen time, simply respond, "Nothing." Be unapologetic about taking breaks or holidays, and if you start to feel worried about being seen as lazy, think of niksen not as a sign of laziness but as an important life skill that might help you regain some composure, find calm, and prevent burnout.

Choose the initial discomfort of niksen over the familiarity of busyness. This might be very hard to do at first. As humans, we want to belong, and when everyone else is hurried and busy, we can be tempted to fall into the same trap.

Tony Crabbe, the author of *Busy*, suggests making use of our social brains and surrounding ourselves with niksen-minded people. Resisting cultural pressures is so much easier when done with others. Or you can do what my mom does and hang a sign on your office door that reads: I BITE. My mom doesn't bite, but it's clear that she doesn't want to be disturbed.

Work and Rest According to Your Natural Rhythm

People have different chronotypes, which means that they need to sleep and work at different times of the day to achieve maximum productivity. Some of us are at our best in the morning, while others feel most productive in the afternoon.

"Everyone of us should figure out when we're at our most creative. Most productive. And niksen is part of this," says Manfred Kets de Vries. He advises drawing a diagram like the one below:

	IMPORTANT	NOT IMPORTANT
LIKE		
DON'T LIKE		

Then look at your activities, tasks, and obligations and decide where they fit on the diagram. You can also use this tool to schedule some niksen time.

"Niksen is recuperating time. *Like* and *not important* — at least from a business point of view. But for your recovery it's very important," explains Kets de Vries. In my opinion, you can call niksen unimportant only if you subscribe to the idea that we should be working all the time.

Depending on what kind of work you do, it may be more difficult to find "niksen niches" in your workday. Remember this: they don't have to be huge pockets of time as long as you make them count. "Everybody has periods of time when they're working by themselves, and we have the ability to control our schedules at least to some degree. So you can take breaks in your own office or your own cubicle," says Pozen. It doesn't have to get any more complicated than taking your eyes off the screen (you can close them if that's easier) and sitting there for a while.

Freelancers like myself are familiar with the feast-orfamine cycle of work, in which we are either overwhelmed or underwhelmed with work. But most work is seasonal, so workers who go into an office every day also deal with periods of heightened and intense work activity and then periods of less activity. It's important for us to be aware of this, because when the tsunami of work comes our way, we're going to have to put more effort into creating pockets of time for niks.

Experiment

For one week, try to respond to every email, message, and notification you receive. As Chris Bailey advises in his book *The Productivity Project,* try working a ninety-hour week. Pull all-nighters and work through the weekend and take absolutely no breaks.

Another week, try the opposite. "Don't have your phone nearby, and when you want to take a break, find something that is pleasurably effortless to do that lets your mind wander a little bit and rest your attention," says Bailey. Then, notice how much energy you have during each of those weeks.

You may not even need to put yourself through this experiment because the results are predictable. Chances are you will find that you feel best on the days when you're not obsessively checking your phone. "Just because something is stimulating doesn't mean that it makes us happy," Bailey says, referring not just to our phones. "I think we need to connect to how these things make us feel."

If you are open to niksen opportunities, I'm sure you'll surprise yourself at how good you can become at doing nothing. Maybe you'll find you already do quite a bit of niks, but now you can do it without feeling guilty about it, knowing that you're doing yourself a favor.

Or you might not even feel like you're doing nothing but simply feel rested or like you've found space to come up with new ideas.

Niksen is a little like learning any other new skill — we're best at it when we come at it playfully and when we're having fun.

Practice Meeting Management

Though work meetings may not be everyone's favorite activity, they are not totally useless. Meetings can be a great way to promote group cohesion and improve cooperation between team members. Meeting face-to-face also makes it possible to read signals that are often missing from electronic communication, such as body language.

In the Netherlands, meetings are important as a tool to create consensus and make sure everyone's voice is heard. They are a crucial part of the decision-making process in this country. But it's important not to ignore the forest for the trees, and not to hold meetings simply because everyone is doing them.

"I advocate shorter meetings. It's hard to take a break when you're in a meeting. And when you're in the third hour, most people have lost attention," says Robert Pozen. In fact, meetings have been found to be one of the reasons

(145)

executives don't get more done. Pozen suggests committing to a maximum of ninety minutes per meeting. (And if you ask me, even that is too long.)

Fight Face Time Culture

Connected to the meeting mentality is face time culture, which expects employees to never leave work before the boss does. "In a lot of American organizations, you're there so the boss can see you," Pozen explains. And as Naoko Yamamoto notices, face time culture is also prevalent in Japan, and undoubtedly in many other countries too.

I experienced something similar years ago when I worked for a translation agency. Sometimes there was no work to be done for hours on end, but I couldn't go home because my contract said that I had to be at work for a certain number of hours every day. Just because you are in the building or even in the line of sight doesn't mean that you are getting things done. You might spend your day secretly playing video games on your computer.

The pressure on employees to be seen working at all times is real. We need to try to change the culture, and it should change from the top. For example, when managers take parental leave, their employees can follow suit. If you are the boss, be an example to your employees. "If you have a team or you're supervising people, you can encourage this culture of taking breaks," says Robert Pozen.

Take regular niksen breaks yourself and be seen doing nothing once in a while. Remember, if you spend day and night at the office, your employees will do the same, but they will follow your lead if you leave work early or take a moment to relax. Focus on the work your team is getting done in a day, week, or month rather than on how many hours your employees are seated behind their computers. And remember: Niksen isn't just good for business. It's humane.

Manage Distractions

Trying to respond to the millions of messages that we get every day, multiple times a day, is a huge distraction from our work or from niksen time. While I agree that email is important in a work-related context, not all emails are necessary for your job, and you shouldn't feel required to respond to every notification that blinks across your screen.

But telling someone to let go of those distractions is "like putting a tray of doughnuts in front of somebody and telling them to resist the urge to smell them and eat them," says Chris Bailey.

If you are someone who constantly feels the urge to grab your phone every time you sit down to do niks, consider the following suggestion. Get yourself a small notebook in which to jot down the thoughts that come up. That way you don't have to rely on your phone, and won't get sucked into browsing Facebook, starting a tweetstorm, or playing Candy Crush. "If you have a really compelling thought that won't let you just sit, write it down and set it aside," suggests Doreen Dodgen-Magee.

(147)

The notebook can also be used for a brain dump. This is a writing technique in which you put to paper everything that is on your mind, from worries that clutter your day to random thoughts, for about five minutes. This will not just clear your thoughts, but also trick the brain into believing you have taken care of these issues. This then frees you to "be present to this moment and just feel," as Dodgen-Magee puts it. Or just niks.

From there we can begin to exercise our niksen muscles and learn to sit with the uncomfortable feelings of boredom and unproductivity. "We have to have that internal locus of control and value ourselves for doing this thing that will make us healthier. Because the world, absolutely, is not going to do that for us," says Dodgen-Magee.

Niksen at Home

For many, home is the place to relax and be yourself. But it can also be a stressful place — for instance, if it's also your place of work, be it paid or unpaid. Home is also where most of your obligations are, even more so if you have a family. As you know from the introduction, sometimes my house talks to me, reminding me of everything I've failed to do. Remember: chores, childrearing, and relationships are all work, so you're just as entitled to breaks as when you're at an office job.

Here are some tips to help you become more comfortable with niksening at home.

Manage Your Expectations

Often, we feel guilty when we're not engaged in some kind of activity that we believe we should be doing. This is generally related to a feeling of not living in accordance with our values.

"I value eating well. So, if I eat an extra-large pizza, I'm going to feel guilty about eating that pizza. I value being healthy and not feeling bloated. Guilt is an informative emotion that might prevent me from doing that thing," explains Chris Bailey.

Taking breaks can also cause feelings of guilt about not working, and that is informative too. "Paradoxically, taking a break makes us feel like we're not living in accordance with our values. We value accomplishing things. We value making a difference. And we value doing what other people expect us to do," Bailey says. But we can easily try to switch that narrative. "We can counter-balance these beliefs by realizing that we value time for reflection. We value having an abundance of energy. We value having presence of mind when we're with our coworkers or when we're with our families."

Doreen Dodgen-Magee thinks reframing the way we think about rest could help us value those quiet moments much more. "When I talk to folks about this, they understand — *Oh, there is value to this,* they say. There is a value to learning to be still and to be present."

Learning takes time and effort, so don't become discouraged if you don't take to niksen immediately. Know that sitting around doing nothing might actually feel un-

(149)

comfortable at first, and that's okay. And it's especially uncomfortable when you have chores or work to do and usually don't wind down 'til you're done.

Doing nothing might feel terrible to the beginner simply because you're a beginner and just not very good at it yet. Don't feel discouraged. Keep at it and see if you start liking it.

Reorganize Your Environment
Before my *New York Times* story, I hadn't thought much about the way our surroundings influence us. I considered niksen a simple matter of willpower and consistency. And while these are important and helpful, having a niksen-friendly space will definitely help you do more sweet, sweet nothing. "If those spaces are present, people will use them," Dodgen-Magee says.

This is known as "nudge theory," popularized by economist Richard Thaler and legal scholar Cass Sunstein in their book *Nudge: Improving Decisions About Health, Wealth, and Happiness,* which describes the way seemingly unimportant decisions such as cafeteria layouts affect our decision-making process. You can make use of that theory and turn your home into a niksen-friendly area. Add a soft couch, a comfy armchair, a few cushions, or just a blanket. These wonderful things might not be necessary, but they're nice and might make you never want to leave your couch ever again. I've read so many articles about making nooks for children to enjoy some quiet time, but that idea is fabulous for adults

(150)

as well. Cozy nooks are fantastic, no matter how old you are.

Choose calming colors like blue or green rather than vivid reds and yellows. Place furniture around a window or a fireplace rather than a TV. This will stimulate not just family time and quietness but also give you more opportunities for niksen. Chances are if we're staring at a TV, it will be only a matter of time before we have the remote in our hands.

Having your space ready for you makes it easier to engage in niksen. You don't have to set anything up or tap into willpower. You can just start. Consider the time you spend picking out the right outfit each morning. Some people, like Mark Zuckerberg or the late Steve Jobs, wear the same thing every day—simply because taking away the dilemma over what to wear frees up time and space for them to make other, maybe more important choices. If you have your niksen space set up in your home, you don't have to spend time thinking about how and where you're going to do it. You just sit down and niks.

I also recommend a little basket or box in your hallway or kitchen where you can put your phone every now and then. If it's always in your hand or in your pocket or just nearby on a table, it's going to tug at you and distract you. So resist that temptation and put that phone away.

(151)

Let Your Children Help
There are so many things to do in the home, and partners can share in those responsibilities equally. But if you have

children they live in your house as well, and after a certain age they can become great helpers. While their chores may take them some time to get used to and they may be slow, they will very quickly become better at what they need to do. And you can help them in surprising ways. For example, we recently threw out many of our children's toys and they didn't complain. Instead, they thanked us for helping them get rid of all that clutter and appreciate that cleaning up now takes them less time.

Less chaos equals less to clean, equals more free time, equals more niksen. Not just for children.

What our children need, says parenting expert Catharina Haverkamp, is a feeling of belonging. They want to know that it's okay for them to be here. "Chores are a perfect way to give our children a sense of responsibility, and it will also make them feel that they belong. They will benefit from the sense of agency it gives them."

Outsource or Let Go
Hiring household help can be a contentious issue because many people feel guilty about employing someone to do what they feel they should be doing themselves.

This is especially true when it comes to childcare. Even the wealthy women described by Wednesday Martin in *Primates of Park Avenue: A Memoir* insisted on taking care of their children themselves while they outsourced practically everything else.

Another way to have others help with your children that I am a big proponent of is daycare. I know this option may not be available to many parents in the US or UK, where this sort of childcare is expensive and there is stigma attached to not being with your child every moment of the day. But I am lucky to be in the Netherlands and able to take advantage of this type of childcare.

It was an amazing experience for us. Every day the nannies invented games and fun activities for my children, who came home with beautiful new artwork and happy faces. The children learned the Dutch language and the local traditions and now feel very much at home in the Netherlands. For that, I'll always be grateful.

Think about what things you want (and can afford) to outsource, how often, and to whom. Then use the time this gives you to work, get some exercise, or, yes, niksen. A while ago, I wrote an article for *O, the Oprah Magazine* in which I shared some advice on how to fight that nagging voice in your head pressuring you to always be doing more. In the article, I suggest asking yourself three questions:

1. Will not doing this task affect your safety, health, or well-being?
2. Is this necessary?
3. Is this my job?

If the answer to any of these questions is yes, go ahead and do it, but you will find that in many cases, the answer to these questions will be a resounding "no."

In my Facebook group, The Nikseneers, someone suggested making a not-to-do-list, and in *The Joy of Doing Nothing: A Real-Life Guide to Stepping Back, Slowing Down, and Creating a Simpler, Joy-Filled Life,* Canadian journalist Rachel Jonat gives the exact same advice. I thought this was a brilliant solution, and it might be even more useful than some to-do lists. The idea is to find things you want to stop doing, then ask yourself whether any of these tasks will help you achieve anything and whether there are any considerable negative consequences associated with not doing this task. Then learn to say no to the tasks that don't move you forward. In the time you free up, you can niks around.

De-schedule Your Kids

It's not just adults who benefit from niksen. Kids do too. Not only does resting or getting bored have benefits for children, it actually affects them more than it does adults because it teaches them from a young age to be more self-reliant and independent. Also, their brains are more adaptive than ours are and the benefits consolidate more quickly. Niksening will teach your children to sit with uncomfortable feelings instead of immediately acting on them.

(154)

"Making more niksen time means setting boundaries around how you spend time, not negating responsibilities that need tending to. How each family sets their boundaries is up to them," says Juli Fraga. Some of her ideas include reducing the number of weekend commitments and scheduling time away for doing nothing.

"Call me lazy, but I have a lot of niksen time on the weekends. I make zero plans, relax on my couch with my favorite blanket and my cat, and enjoy observing the thoughts that travel through my mind," Juli Fraga says. Some may call this spacing out, but Fraga prefers to call it tuning in. To her, the benefits are visible right away.

"Doing nothing isn't 'nothing,' and it can end up being an enormous something when we see how pulling back on busyness can bolster our physical and emotional health," she adds.

Giving children the experience of doing niks, and letting them create and imagine what to do with that time, isn't optional, "it's a required experience for a child," believes Tony Crabbe, who calls boredom the greatest gift he can give his children.

Be a Role Model

"Parents can be leaders in this doing nothing, niksen," Catharina Haverkamp says. If we can't do it for our own sake, maybe we can think of our children. We need niksen, but they do too.

And Tony Crabbe agrees. "Children see parents' behavior as social proof of what's right. If children see parents on their phones all the time, then children follow that route as well. That is role modeling," he explains.

Start by teaching children to entertain themselves. Let

(155)

them hang around, give them permission to be lazy, don't solve all their problems, give life a chance to just be lived, trust, and rest. "When they don't know what to do, they just don't know what to do, that's it," says Haverkamp.

This, of course, is very hard to do. Critics may even accuse us of neglecting our children, but nothing could be further from the truth. And we can even learn from our kids, who may be better at niksen than we are.

"My son takes a shower. And he gets out of the shower and then he doesn't get dressed, he just sits there in the towel and sits there singing for half an hour. That's niksen, isn't it?" fellow writer Michele Hutchison asks me. If you ask me, this, exactly this, is the very soul of niksen, and we can all learn from her son.

I know sometimes there is nothing more frustrating than seeing your child do nothing while you need to do laundry and unload the dishwasher and cook dinner and sweep the floors. But if the kids have performed their duties, such as homework or chores, let them be, and give yourself a break too.

Do Nothing, Together

I always thought of niksen as something that you do alone in your home, by yourself. But those sweet nothing moments can become more special when they are shared. Crabbe calls this "the niksen of togetherness" and it could be "a great way to find out what it means to genuinely do nothing while with somebody else."

This reminds me of something psychologist Doreen

Dodgen-Magee told me: She encourages people to host boredom parties, at which a host invites over a few friends to be bored together.

There will always be moments of silence in a conversation. And it can be important and also very rewarding to be able to do nothing together. "That notion of being comfortable enough to sit quietly with somebody . . . You could watch the sunset," Crabbe says.

For many parents, the best thing in the world can be reading to their children or playing with them. To me, it's hugging. Sometimes, when I'm in a great mood, I'll ask, "Who wants a hug?" And if I'm lucky, at least one of the three kids will be willing to put their little arms around me and give me a cuddle. Sometimes, I'll lie down with them on the floor and do nothing but just put my arms around them. The fact that they are small and soft and smell good definitely helps.

Many of you might not have children but may instead have huggable animals such as cats or dogs. When your cat sits on your lap and prevents you from doing anything, use that as an excuse for niksen.

When the kids are in bed, my husband and I often watch a TV series together. I'm usually snuggled into my husband because he is soft and warm and has his arm around me, and I often think that the series is secondary. I'm simply niksening up against him.

(157)

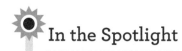

In the Spotlight

Equal Division of Labor

Lisa is an American living in Sweden with her husband, Jon, and their two children, ages six and eight.

They say the division of household labor has morphed over time to take on an "if you see it, do it" type approach with only a few exceptions.

Jon loves delicious food. With time, he discovered that while Lisa has many skills, they do not extend into the kitchen. "He loves to test new recipes, buy spices, and try out exotic flavors . . ." Since she's "just as happy eating pasta with a boring red sauce as he is eating a fragrant Thai curry with coconut rice," the meal preparations are Jon's domain.

They both try to be actively involved in their kids' school lives. They split drop-off and pick-up, with Jon dropping them off in the mornings on his way to work. Lisa picks them up after school and is generally the parent who attends the after-school meetings, dances, and extracurricular activities.

Not everything is split 50-50 between them, but they do try to balance their home and work lives. For example, since Lisa works from home as a freelancer, she doesn't socialize so much on a daily basis with friends or colleagues. Jon and Lisa both know that leaving the house daily is essential for their mental health, so Jon often adapts his work schedule to get home early so that

(158)

Lisa can head out for her volunteer activities, dinners with friends, or other types of social activities. In return, Lisa makes space for Jon to go out for a guys' night about once a month so he also gets some downtime outside of the house and the office.

Niksen Out in Public

I do not consider public spaces to be very niksen friendly. After all, you go out with the specific purpose of either becoming active, like in the case of sports, or socializing. Or maybe you're taking your children to one of their many after-school activities. Or maybe you've taken up yoga or ceramics. And the public is, sadly, very lacking in blankets, comfy armchairs, and, especially, couches. But keep in mind that the public space offers many opportunities for niksen if you know how to spot them.

Sports . . . but with Niksen in Mind
While Americans may go for a spin class and the Dutch will jump on an actual bike, sports are important on both sides of the Atlantic. With our lives becoming more and more sedentary, physical activities have become vital if we don't want to compromise our health and well-being. But niksen is also vital to our health and well-being.

(159)

You don't have to go to the gym or a yoga class every day. And you don't have to spend hours there to reap the benefits of exercise. If you enjoy spending hours jogging, by all means, continue to do just that. The World Health Organization's guidelines recommend thirty minutes a day, five days a week. That's reasonable, I think.

But while you're out running, playing tennis, or taking a spin class, remember to sneak in a little niksen time here and there. "When I run, my gaze is focused in the distance and my mind can wander. Often, I'm struck by the beauty of my surroundings," says Pam Moore, a writer who coaches women interested in running. If it weren't for the running, I would have sworn she was talking about niksen.

Just like Moore, you could pick a niksen-friendly type of sport and build niksen into your exercise regime. She leaves her phone at home when she runs and does not listen to any music or podcasts. "On the few occasions that I have listened to something, I've felt disconnected from my breathing and from my body and I didn't enjoy running as much," she says.

Find a Niksen-Friendly Hobby

Hobbies bring us into a state of flow and help us relax, allowing us to do or create something that is not work and not in service of the family. Niksen can fit seamlessly into that definition. "I'd say hobbies are important in life because they offer a break from the rest of our life. Look for hobbies that take your mind off that which you're usually doing," says writer Mary Widdicks.

Take it from Widdicks, who used to care for freshwater aquariums. That hobby started out as a project for her children but then turned into something more. "The aquarium was this unexpectedly complex and ordered world that I could tend to. It followed rules. It made sense. And that was unbelievably calming among the crazy that is a house filled with three children. The sense of self-efficacy was extremely comforting, like slowly tuning a dial," she tells me. "There were nights after my kids went to bed when I'd make a cup of tea, turn off all the lights except the tank lights, and just watch the fish. If you watched long enough, it became clear that the fish had their own social structure and territories."

Moreover, after learning she was prone to overmanaging the aquarium, she backed off and observed a little more and did a little less. And the balance came back. "Sometimes the best thing to do is nothing," she says. I couldn't agree more.

Go Niks Someplace Else

Lots of freelancers like to work at a nice café because it can be hard to concentrate at home. The laundry beckons, the dishes in the sink glare at you, and it's hard to ignore their call and just work.

The same can be said of niksen. Even though we probably instinctively think of the home when considering where to relax, the truth is that for many of us our homes can actually be stress inducing.

The solution: get out of there. A café can be a great place to sit down with a cup of hot coffee or tea and a brownie or a croissant. You'll feel more unencumbered because someone else is responsible for keeping the space around you clean and you have almost no responsibilities in a place like that. You even have people running around entirely devoted to bringing you hot or cold beverages of your choice and sweet or salty snacks.

"The café, especially my favorite one, kills so many birds with one stone. It is set along a beach and it has two floors. And the view and the sea air are priceless," says Pinar Tarhan, a writer and friend of mine based in Istanbul, Turkey. Pinar has ADHD, so it's hard for her to really sit down and do niks. But even she gets some niksen time while working at her favorite café.

"I'm constantly moving to get coffee or to take a break. I people watch and I listen. I also take pictures. There are moments when I just do nothing and sip my coffee," she tells me. And she loves it when the café plays music at a low volume. "Just existing in a calm environment without too much noise and a great view is beyond relaxing and rewarding," she says.

Nature, too, offers great opportunities for niksen. Go to the park, find yourself a nice bench or a comfy spot in the grass or under a tree, and sit down. Watch the birds fly by and check out the people in the park walking their dogs. Notice the trees and the weather and the squirrels and other animals.

By choosing an outdoorsy space such as the park or the beach, you get the additional benefits of being outside, which are really good for you. You can combine niksen with a daily walk or your jogging routine. Remember, there is no wrong way to do this—just unplug for a while.

Learn to Live at Two Speeds

When Tony Crabbe was young, he used to play Ping-Pong with his brother, and they prided themselves on their ability to play really fast. "One day I played against a guy who could play fast too," remembers Crabbe. But the man also knew how to slow the ball down, on purpose. He beat Crabbe with ease. "I think we need to learn the art of adjusting our pace intentionally," he says. This is a great example of how switching gears from fast to slow can help us win—in both the literal and the metaphorical senses of the word.

Matthieu Boisgontier, a therapist and researcher on inactivity, tells me about the cognitive switch. He uses it to motivate people to become more active, but it can work for niksen as well. "To decide that we're going to sit and do nothing, we need cognition. And we need cognition to say, 'and now I want to be physically active because it's good for my health.' Cognition is how you make the switch in a situation," explains Boisgontier.

Cognition requires conscious thought. "We should be able to decide what we are going to do and not just follow our automatic habits. People should be able to switch their brain on and say, 'No no no! I want to be more physically active, I want to take the stairs,'" says Boisgontier.

And it's similar with niksen. "When you are doing millions of things at the same time, there is Twitter, there are

(163)

emails, there is work. You should be able to switch and say, 'I'm not working efficiently anymore. I should take one hour to rest. And I will come back to the work after that.' You get to a point where you need this switch to change your situation, and this is cognition," he explains.

On a side note, I'm not advocating an empty life (although many of us would love that). A busy life can be a fulfilling, happy life. But we need to be able to slow down consciously at times too. You won't know whether niksen is the way for you until you try it. "Being happy is a matter of trial and error; try some ways to niksen and see how you like it," recommends sociologist Ruut Veenhoven.

In the Spotlight

Two Ways to Niks

I've found that if you want more niksen time, you have two options:

1. Plan It
The first approach is that you plan chunks of time with the very specific purpose of doing nothing. Just think about it. You make time for things like going to the gym, or work, or to be with your family, all of which we consider to be important.

But somehow, in the whirlwind of duties and responsibilities, we forget to schedule time for ourselves and for doing nothing. We run from one activity to the next, and we seem unable to stop running.

If that's you, then it's time to say, "Hey, wait a minute. What am I doing?"

It's time to treat your niksen time as one of the most important things on Earth. Your mental and physical health matter, and niksen will boost both of those.

It's time to choose niksen with conscious effort. Sometimes this will mean you need to schedule niksen instead of other activities that might seem more interesting, exciting, or important. Jenny Odell, author of *How to Do Nothing,* calls this NOMO, or necessity of missing out. You can put niksen on your agenda. Or even better, as Laura Vanderkam advises in *Off the Clock: Feel Less Busy While Getting More Done,* leave some white space in your agenda. That will make your other appointments so much more prominent but not overwhelm you.

2. Go Out and Find It

The alternative to scheduling time for doing nothing is actively welcoming niksen as it shows up in your daily life. Consider all the situations in which you're used to grabbing your phone and scrolling through a Twitter feed or some other social media. When you start to see the world through niksen-tinted glasses, you'll find plenty of opportunities for niksen — for instance, while you're waiting for something or taking a break.

"For example, if you have ten minutes or if you're waiting for your kids to come back from school or the

(165)

playground, instead of getting your phone out to swipe and scroll the boredom away, you could stare into space. Stare at the clouds, smell the coffee. Just let your mind wander," says Sandi Mann.

Mann loves to use her commute as niksen time, and she tells me she doesn't turn the radio on, just so that her mind is free to wander. We should grab every opportunity we get for niksen. "Standing in line at the supermarket, don't get out your phone, just look around, daydream," she says.

Pick your favorite way to niks depending on your schedule, needs, and personality.

Wrapping It Up

This chapter discussed how you can introduce niksen into your own life's most important areas: work, home, and the public space. Some ideas include taking breaks with purpose, redefining productivity, and fighting productivity pressure. At home, it is important that chores are shared by all family members so that everyone can enjoy niksen time, and it's a good idea to have a niksen space, like a nook, that you can settle into easily. In the public space, you can find hobbies that can be combined with niksen and do sports with niksen in mind. Now you can choose ways to niks that suit your personality and personal circumstances.

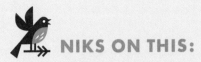

NIKS ON THIS:

. . . .

- What steps can you take to introduce niksen into your own life?

- Which areas of your life discussed in this chapter need more niksening up?

- When do you think you should speed up or slow down?

(167)

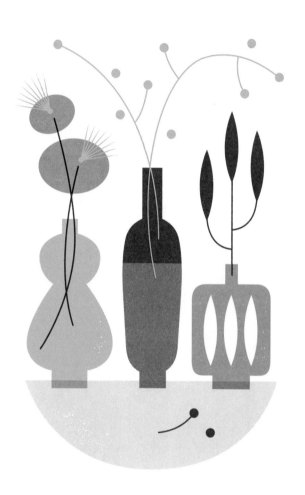

When Niksen
Doesn't Work

I'm on my couch and yet again, I think: *Niksen is great and I love it, but will it work for everyone?* Chances are it won't. And I can think of several situations in which niksen would be a very, very bad idea. So how are we supposed to know when niksen is okay and when it isn't?

Once again, consider the following three scenarios.

1. I'm on my couch. I'm slumped into my pillows and have no desire to do anything. I have not been exercising, working, or present with my kids. There is a mountain of laundry to be taken care of, dinner won't make itself, and I've been eating way too much chocolate. I have not talked to another adult besides my husband in ages. Nothing is exciting anymore, and I feel like I might have a case of the blues. I'm tired, but this is not my usual, delicious energizing downtime. This is something else.

2. Again, I'm on the couch. I'm happy and ready to get to work. I feel like I can take on anything! I feel challenged in my work, and I'm going to meet a friend in about half an hour. I wonder if I shouldn't be niksening a little more than I do? Am I getting caught up in another whirlwind of activity and busyness? I know how it works. One day, I meet a friend and work on an assignment and there is some time for niks. And the next day, I'm doing all that plus I'm taking care of a sick child, putting out fires, and then some. I end up dropping activities because I just can't take care of everything. Right now, I feel so good, this level of busyness is just right for me. But what about tomorrow? How will I feel then?

3. I'm on the coach, and again, there is a mountain of duties to take care of. There is, there was, and there always will be laundry to wash, a house to clean, children to raise, dinners to make. But I just wish someone else would take care of all of it for a while so I can just sit here on the couch and do nothing all day long. If only someone else could do everything. Wouldn't that be the dream? To have no duties, no obligations, nothing to do? I wish someone would fly in and do it all for me.

In which of these scenarios do you think niksen would be the best solution? Would it surprise you to know that the answer is: none of them?

Why Niksen Might Not Work for All of Us

"Wait," my husband said when I told him what this chapter would be about. "But I thought your book was pro-niksen?"

"It is pro-niksen," I replied, "but terms and conditions apply."

Niksen might not work for you, no matter how hard you try. And even if it has worked well in the past or might work well in the future, there will be moments when it might not be the right path for you.

"Some people are naturally hard-charging, and they like to be busy all the time. And it's hard for them to kick back. They naturally slide into a little activity, like they're going to quickly do a puzzle, or they'll pick up some knitting. Or maybe they're going to catch up on *Game of Thrones*. They might feel these things are a bit of a project while others would see it more as goofing off," Gretchen Rubin tells me.

If you read and believe most wellness books and articles, you might notice that many will argue there is only one way to happiness and that it is their way. Nothing could be further from the truth. "There is no best way to be creative, there is no best way to be happy. We all have to examine our lives for ourselves. And let's say you find relationships are important to you, then how do you do relationships in a way that's right for you? And that's going to look very, very different for each of us," Gretchen Rubin explains.

(171)

Why Culture Matters

It has been shown that cultural, political, and economic circumstances affect child-rearing practices. In their book *Love, Money, and Parenting: How Economics Explains the Way We Raise Our Kids,* Matthias Doepke and Fabrizio Zilibotti argue that parenting choices actually change depending on our economic circumstances and the culture that we live in. It is safe to assume these same circumstances do not only impact our parenting but are also likely to impact how we relax, express happiness, or spend our time.

Sometimes, no matter what you do, wellness trends adopted from other cultures don't work because they are deeply embedded in the culture from which they originate. This is why niksen won't work if it's not supported by the culture in the broadest sense of that word. *Culture* has many definitions but my favorite one is "the way we do things around here." A little less simply put: culture is a way of life — or the behaviors, beliefs, values, and symbols — that a group of people accept, generally without thinking about it, and that are passed along by communication and imitation from one generation to the next.

Kari Leibowitz, a psychology researcher who studies happiness in Norway, thinks we focus too much on the individual level of culture rather than taking a broader perspective.

Wellness books and philosophies have the potential to initiate change at a broader level though. Examples from countries with good welfare systems could show Americans what a welfare society might look like. Irina Dumitrescu, the medieval researcher living in Germany, wonders if they might inspire people in leadership positions to ask themselves: "Are there ways I can help change the culture here? If I have employees, can I try to normalize new values to benefit them?"

Like many of the experts quoted in this book, Dumitrescu finds it extremely problematic that so much wellness and parenting advice focuses on individuals and the choices that they should make. "You can't change your life without having some kind of structure around you. In Germany, when I get sick and want to come in to work, my colleagues will chew me out for that. People in Germany take sick days when they need to and this makes it possible for me to do that too," she says. In many other cultures, it is considered good form to show up to work even when you're sick. The US, for instance, isn't as lenient toward sick employees as many European countries are.

This is why, as Leibowitz says, we can always learn from other cultures, but "you can never do another culture 100 percent because it's embedded in that particular setting. For example, it's easy to love the winter in a country where homelessness isn't a problem and there aren't people freezing to death on the streets," she explains of her experiences in northern Norway.

Different cultures also have different ideas about what appropriate behavior is. Americans tend to value high-arousal positive emotions more than many Europeans, including the Dutch. "Americans really like excitement and joy and feeling good. And they want to feel good in a really upbeat way," she explains. So it might be hard to bring niksen or hygge into this culture. "You can try to implant this European idea of coziness into an American setting, but will this idea take root where running around and being excited is synonymous with feeling good?"

At the individual level, change can come relatively quickly—it is easier to change your own behavior than your whole culture. And there could be a more insidious reason, too, for the popularity of trends from other countries. According to Leibowitz, organizations and the people in power don't always want to stop placing the responsibility for change on individuals.

"I think it's a problem when these foreign cultural concepts are treated like Band-Aids, like substitutes for good infrastructure or supportive communities," Leibowitz tells me.

She notes, for instance, that in the US people feel guilty when they are not able to follow such trends due to work schedules not giving them that space. In America, "it's not an option to say, 'I'm going to sleep more during the winter and come in to work a little later.'" The culture won't allow it.

(174)

Gretchen Rubin agrees that not all trends work in all settings. But she says: "It's good to have many different approaches, because if something doesn't work, well, there is nothing wrong with you, you can just try the next thing on the list. There are many possibilities." Rubin is a firm believer that there is no one right way to happiness or to a good life. And so am I.

Different Things for Different People

Niksen is not only affected by the culture that we are a part of, it is also affected by our personalities. And niksen will not work in identical ways for everyone. For example, Rubin likes to use niksen to stop herself from procrastinating, but that might not work at all for someone else. "If you are a person who has a rich inner life that you can occupy yourself with, this won't work for you, because you can easily spend three hours lost in your own thoughts," she explains. As I listen to her, I admit to myself that I am certainly one of those people.

Niksen is "a tool for a certain kind of person with a certain kind of mind. If it doesn't work, then you have to find a different solution," she tells me.

Niksen is a tool that you can use regularly, keep on standby for when you need it, or discard entirely because it doesn't seem to work for you. It's up to you.

And even productivity experts may struggle with niksen, so you wouldn't be the only one. "I struggle with focus. I struggle with the guilt of taking breaks. And I think that anybody who pretends not to—that's just bullshit. Nothing bugs me more than a productivity expert who pretends to be perfectly productive all the time. Or a happiness expert who pretends to be perfectly happy all the time," says Chris Bailey, the productivity expert. So, let me admit this to you: this niksen expert struggles with niksen too.

Don't Do Niks If . . .

Just like any other trend, niksen may not work for everyone. Moreover, it has become clear from my research that niksen is simply not a good idea in some circumstances. So, if you recognize yourself in any of these situations, consider a different solution.

You're Depressed

Often those suffering from depression have very little energy and may struggle just to get out of bed, which can be counterproductive.

When she became depressed after the death of her daughter, Christy Wilson says, "everyone said *do something.* And I really just wanted to stay in bed and sleep." Still, she and her husband traveled from the US, where they lived, to Europe to visit her sister. "While it was nice to get away and paste a fake smile on our faces, we were both grieving and dying inside," she says.

Yet she never sat still during her depression. "Getting out and being involved in something gave me a sense of purpose and motivation to have a life, find my identity," she says. Niksen would not have helped her then, she believes.

Christy is now a mom of three (and one in heaven) and enjoys her niksen time when she can. She admits that "it took constantly being busy and moving to save myself from that depression, and that taught me to appreciate what doing nothing means . . . When depression strikes and you want to crawl into a hole, the first step should be to ask yourself what in your life is weighing so heavily on your shoulders? The next step is to get up, get moving, exercise, volunteer, spend time with friends (even if you have to plaster a fake smile on your face), and just be present."

In her stress center, Carolien Hamming helps people with stress and burnout, though not necessarily by teaching them to do nothing. Instead, she focuses on slow movement and breathing exercises that are good for the body. It has been shown that a healthy, calm body affects the state of the mind and helps it calm down too.

"Niksen wouldn't work for people in the midst of burnout. Your heart rate is too fast, you're feeling fretful," explains Hamming. "You need to re-regulate your body."

She sees niksen as a way to prevent burnout rather than as a cure for it. "Niksen is for people who are healthy but lead busy lives. It can help them realize that they don't have to be active at all times. But once things are severely out of balance, niksen isn't a solution."

So if you suffer from depression or find yourself with a case of burnout, niksen may not be such a good idea. "Maybe it's better to mess around with a scrapbook, or to keep your body moving," she explains.

It Could Get You in Trouble

You might work at a job where you're constantly monitored. In such cases, doing nothing could have serious repercussions for you. You risk being reprimanded or even fired. This is not a risk worth taking if you need to pay rent and keep your family fed and clothed. If inactivity at work has serious consequences for you, then maybe you don't want to put everything on the line for nothing (literally).

Maybe you've read about the benefits of niksen and wish you could make it fit into your own life, but you can't. If that's the case, don't worry. If it's just not right for you right now, that's fine. There will always be moments when work becomes busy and more stressful or your children get sick or your priorities shift. That is just the way life is, and there will be times when there is just no time for niksen. And that's okay too; you can always niks later.

When There Is Nothing Wrong with Your Life

You know when you go to the doctor with a nagging feeling and vague complaints, only to be told that there is absolutely nothing wrong with you? It's possible the doctor missed important warning signs and you actually have a serious illness. But more likely, it's because there is actually nothing wrong with you.

Sometimes I read a self-help or a parenting book hoping it will help me find a better way of raising my children or living my life, only to realize that I don't really need to change anything and that my life is just fine. Not perfect, but good enough.

You might feel the same way. If that's the case, that's great, because it means that you like your life as it is and don't want to change it. I'm happy for you because — congratulations — maybe you've discovered how to live a happy, fulfilled life, free of stress and challenges.

Even if your job is stressful, and even if you sometimes feel exhausted or overwhelmed by the busyness of daily life, I am sure you can find other — maybe more active — ways to deal with the stress. That's great.

Your experience of busyness and stress is personal, which means that what looks like a pretty relaxed life may be the epitome of boredom to someone else, and what seems exciting and thrilling to you might feel terrifying and overwhelming to someone else.

If you know there's stress in your life but you can deal with it and you feel fulfilled and happy, then maybe you don't need niksen. In the words of Ruut Veenhoven, "Don't take medicine if there is no disease."

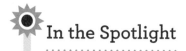

In the Spotlight

....

Flow Experiences

In his famous book *Flow: The Psychology of Optimal Experience*, Hungarian-American psychologist Mihaly Csikszentmihalyi describes an experience he calls "flow" that happens when you are engaged in a meaningful activity. Think of a musician completely disappearing in his music, or a painter so absorbed in her work that she loses track of time. The flow state includes several elements:

- intense and focused concentration on the present moment
- the merging of action and awareness
- a loss of reflective self-consciousness
- a sense of personal control or agency over the situation or activity
- a distortion of temporal experience
- the altering of one's subjective experience of time
- the experience of the activity as intrinsically rewarding

Activities that allow for flow have clearly defined guidelines, offer immediate feedback, and allow their participants to apply skills while simultaneously challenging themselves. "Because of the way they are constructed, they help participants and spectators achieve an ordered state of mind that is highly enjoyable," writes Csikszentmihalyi.

Games, sports, and playing an instrument are a few examples of flow-inducing activities. Crafts, cooking, and other handicrafts could also become flow experiences, as could more intellectual work such as writing. The activity should be neither too hard (which could result in frustration) nor too easy (which can bring on boredom).

A flow-friendly culture provides ample options for flow activity as well as meaningful work opportunities and plenty of leisure time to pursue one's interests.

Is the Netherlands a flow-friendly culture? I believe so, and Csikszentmihalyi agrees. Moreover, many of the things the Dutch do — engaging in sports, cycling to work, hanging out for *gezelligheid* with friends — are perfectly suited to induce flow.

If this appeals to you more than niksen, go for it and pick up a paintbrush. And the best part: it turns out that flow experiences make people just as happy as doing nothing.

How to Cheat Your Brain into Doing Niks

Some people find it hard to do nothing and would rather occupy their hands and minds with a specific activity. If this is you, I have a solution. It involves a little bit of cheating because you're not literally doing nothing, but these niksen "hacks" are simple and flexible.

Listen to Music

When I have to work, my brain can sometimes get in the way by offering thoughts and comments, such as "Hey, did you do the laundry? There is that cooking video that you must check out immediately. And have you looked for a new toaster yet?" I have found that listening to music works wonders in allowing me to concentrate.

Listening to music can have beneficial effects on your well-being and calm you down — or it can give you the energy you need to get up and get to work. And while you're listening to music, you can trick yourself into thinking you're doing something when you're actually not doing much, or to put it the other way around: that you're not doing anything when you are actually listening to music. That's why I like to call it harmless cheating.

"Music," Mihaly Csikszentmihalyi writes in *Flow*, "helps organize the mind that attends to it, and therefore reduces psychic entropy." Psychic entropy is a state of mind, first described by Carl Jung and later discussed by Csikszentmihalyi, characterized by constantly looping negative thought patterns, which leaves us with a reduced ability to deal with external tasks or even inner reflection. We all know the feeling: frazzled, overwhelmed, or paralyzed by worry, and unable to take a break. According to Csikszentmihalyi, music is an antidote to this.

You can, of course, listen to the lyrics and sing along. But if you already know the song by heart, why not listen to the other voices and the instruments that aren't as obvious and try to follow their melodies? Or try doing what a friend of mine does: "When I concentrate really hard, I can sometimes hear all the instruments separately." Try to separate the violins from the cellos, the trumpets from the saxophones, and the flutes from the oboes. Listening like this can trick your brain into a state of niksen — you may find yourself letting go of your daily concerns.

Create Something

In 2017, adult coloring books were all the rage. Experts touted the benefits of coloring, saying it was great for our mental health and it allowed us to focus on a simple but rewarding activity while letting our minds wander a little.

It turns out that when you can distract yourself from your usual preoccupations, you can relax. This might be why so many people love knitting; the clickety-clack of the needles is relaxing and helps minds wander. Well, isn't that what niksen is all about?

It doesn't really matter if you're cooking, painting, crocheting, or scrapbooking. The important thing is that you remove yourself from the busyness of real life for a while in a way that doesn't require much brain space, so that you can reap the benefits of niksen while you're at it. Repetitive activities like coloring or knitting work best, but each of us should find what feels good.

(183)

"Activities that allow a small amount of cognitive load to be used free the rest of the mind up. You use your mind just enough so you don't get bored. A good activity is one that you need to pay a little attention to, but not one that's too exciting. Coloring or knitting work well," explains Sandi Mann, the British psychologist who studies the benefits of boredom.

And as an extra bonus, when we create something tangible and beautiful in the process of distracting ourselves, we also boost our self-esteem.

Play!

I could watch marble runs and dominos fall for hours. There is something extremely satisfying about those steady, repetitive movements. But when adults play like kids, it is usually frowned upon. Society reprimands the playful adult: "You're not a child anymore." The only play that's accepted is competitive, as in the case of sports.

Like rest, play and playfulness are very important to our well-being. They are also a little bit rebellious — and in that sense, just like niksen.

Play should be engaged in without a specific purpose in mind. We don't play to feel better or to think more creatively. That's strategy, not play. Play starts with curiosity and ends somewhere unexpected, but with enhanced feelings of well-being and creativity.

Psychologist Doreen Dodgen-Magee encourages her adult clients to use toys such as kinetic sand or stress balls.

These keep our hands occupied while our minds are free to wander. Many people feel calmer when touching or squeezing toys (that's what stress balls are for, after all), and this can help relieve their stress and anxiety. Lego has seen the potential in that and started making sets aimed at adults. Recently, there has also been increased interest in games. And not necessarily just video games but old-fashioned board games too.

You don't need toys to play: you could try little mind games too. Make them up; there are no rules. I do it a lot. When I'm faced with a boring task like watching my children at the playground, I play a game in my mind. I count the seconds and try to get to five minutes. I can only briefly look at my phone to see if my timing is on point. Often, I'm right, but sometimes I'm too fast and sometimes I'm too slow. But that doesn't matter; it's just a game I play to occupy myself. I'm not trying to achieve anything.

When I do this, time passes faster and I don't feel as bored. And I often find my mind wandering and coming up with ideas. It helps bring my mind into that alert and creative state.

If you're bored, turn whatever you're doing into a game, just like kids do. If you're trying to niks, you can make a game out of that. How many minutes can you do it for? Five? Good, try ten! You can sit still with a stress ball? Awesome, but can you do it without one? Playfully challenge yourself.

Go for a Walk

Manfred Kets de Vries tells me that he likes to take long walks during his work breaks. They help him focus, and he finds them very calming. The park is his favorite place to go, but there are many other places he happily walks in too. The surroundings don't matter so much; it's the repetitive movement and the rhythm of his steps that are calming.

You can take walks anywhere, the city included. Songs and poems have been written about the *flaneur*, someone who walks around a city with no goal other than walking, watching people, and admiring buildings. As much as I love urban environments, science shows that walking in nature is preferable and has greater benefits for your mental and physical health.

I've had many of my greatest ideas while walking in the dunes or in the forest with my family.

Ride Your Bike

In the Netherlands, people don't cycle just for pleasure or for health benefits. A bicycle is an actual form of transportation to bring people from A to B quickly and efficiently. It is as important in the Netherlands as a car is in the US.

Because the Dutch are practically one with their two-wheelers, they don't consider cycling to be an effort at all. They are so used to being on bicycles that they can just let their legs push the pedals and let their minds wander.

If you've ever biked competitively or treated your bicycling like a sport, try a slower pace, and don't worry about the kilometers or miles or how many calories you've burned. Just let the movement take over and allow your mind to wander.

Listen to Your Body

Doreen Dodgen-Magee suggests a technique known as grounding, which includes focusing on your five senses to get you out of your head and into your body. It is similar to niksen and it might even give you the feeling that you're being mindful.

"*How does the air feel on my skin? Or how does the weight of my body feel on this chair? What do I smell?* It's not creating a moment, but just bringing oneself fully present to the moment," explains Dodgen-Magee.

Sometimes, instead of niksening, I ask myself, "How am I feeling at this given moment?" and then I try to scan my body for answers. Am I hungry? Thirsty? Hot? Cold? This is important because it prevents meltdowns when I get hangry. If you're not familiar with this term, it's a portmanteau of the words *hungry* and *angry*. You know how you sometimes want to murder someone but feel much better after eating a pizza? That's hanger.

Listening to the body allows for interoception, a process by which our brains or minds make sense of the signals coming from the body. Disrupted interoception is now known to play a part in mood and anxiety disorders. So, taking some time to sit and understand the body's signals is a great way to spend time. If niksen is not for you, maybe this will work better.

Wrapping It Up

When I ask Gretchen Rubin why most wellness trends are so rigid, she says, "We'd all be fixed if there was just one way and we could figure it out. People just want one answer. They want you to tell them to go into nature for 120 minutes a week and breathe deeply eight times, and that's it. People feel it's simpler if they are given a very clear blueprint, whereas in real life there is much more room to wiggle."

In this chapter you've learned about situations in which niksen doesn't work and what to do instead. For example, if you suffer from depression, it might be more beneficial to focus on slowly getting up and about and getting help instead of niksening (although I also acknowledge that there are times in depression when you can't move, and that's fine too). Another reason niksen might not be for you is if you don't want to change anything about your life.

We also went through some little tricks to cheat your brain into niksening while you're actually doing something, like listening to music or playing, and there are some suggestions about what to do instead of niksening, like listening to your body.

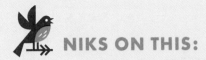

NIKS ON THIS:

· ·

- Can you think of situations when you wanted to do niks but instead got active in some way and that helped more?

- What is your favorite way to relax?

- Are you the type of person who can do niks easily?

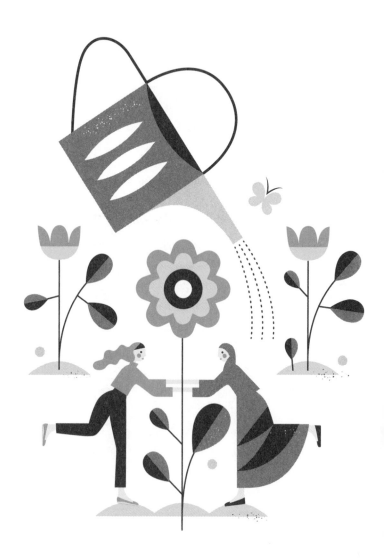

Creating Nikstopia

For the last time in this book, I'm on my couch, now pondering all the ways niksen has changed my life. It has taken a while, but I have finally arrived. I have somehow managed to soak up all the goodness that niksen has to offer, and now my life is a constant niksen-fest.

My house cleans itself while I lie on my coach and occasionally read a book and drink a cup of tea (old habits die hard). The laundry also takes care of itself, singing happy songs while it pulls itself out of the washing machine, hangs itself on the drying rack, and later folds itself neatly into our wardrobes.

Every day I wake up happy and relaxed, looking forward to all the niksen I'm going to enjoy that day. I'm never angry. I'm never tired. After all, if you're experiencing any kind of negative emotion during your niksening practice, you're doing it wrong! And since I have perfected the Dutch art of doing nothing, I have perfected myself. Just try it, and success will be yours. Stop whatever you're doing, and everything will fall into place.

You don't believe me, do you? I certainly hope not, because once again, I made that all up.

The truth is that I still feel overwhelmed by pretty much everything. I still feel like I can't handle it all. I still want to ask my mom, the genetics professor, to clone me so I'd have some help around here. She is refusing, but wouldn't it be nice to have several Olgas to help take care of things?

And when I finally do find some free time, I rarely spend all of it on niksen. In fact, that's usually when I am reminded of all the things I still have to do.

I was, I am, and I probably always will be a mess. Thanks to my magnetic board I no longer forget my appointments, so that's an improvement, but otherwise, I walk around the world in a constant state of confusion. And I still lack the deep well of patience and emotional control that Dutch parents seem to master naturally.

You must be wondering, *Why is this the person trying to teach me how to niks? What does this joker know that I don't?*

I may have started this book with a joke and now again shared some of my own personal failures in this domain, but niksen is no joke. I believe that niksen is about much more than our personal busyness. Its message is bigger and far more important than that. Let's take a peek into the future to put it into perspective, and after that we'll see what we can really achieve, on a large scale, with niksen.

What Will the Future Bring? Robots, Stress, and More Busyness!

According to Tony Crabbe in *Busy*, we're not going to become less overwhelmed anytime soon. "It's not your fault," he says somewhat reassuringly. In fact, we might even become busier still, despite robots and AI taking over some of our jobs. This same advancing technology will demand even more of our attention, leading to more overwhelm. And that technology is becoming more and more sophisticated too, which will make unplugging and doing nothing much more difficult.

What concerns me most are the growing levels of stress and the fact that burnout is becoming more common, especially among Millennials. This stress is related to the growing economic instability that we are faced with, increased health care costs, and the climate crisis. Some people now suffer from climate change–related anxiety, known as eco-anxiety. These are serious issues that need our attention immediately.

I'm not telling you this to depress you. I actually believe that the time has come for us to start imagining a better

(193)

world, a thriving world. As Dutch historian Rutger Bregman points out in *Utopia for Realists: How We Can Build the Ideal World,* many of the freedoms and privileges we take for granted today used to be no more than ideas in a bright person's mind. In fact, he writes, "Ideas that seem politically impossible may one day become politically inevitable." And they all start with a question: What if . . . ?

What If . . .

In *From What Is to What If,* writer and environmentalist Rob Hopkins describes a utopia and provides examples of neighborhoods that produce their own food and create spaces for children to play and run wild. He talks about schools that foster the power of imagination and ethical banks and workplaces. His vision seems unreal, especially at the beginning, but the projects he describes are fully based in reality.

Utopia may not be as far away as we think. There are several niksen-friendly places in the world already, including the Netherlands. I have spun my own vision of a niksen-friendly future and I'd like to share it with you. And it reaches far beyond "just" doing nothing. What follows are several ideas for a Nikstopia. What if . . .

We Redefined Productivity

It is time that we collectively redefine productivity so that niksen has a place in that definition. Being productive is not only a matter of how hard or how long we work. It's not even about our accomplishments. We need to let go of the idea that our worth is connected to some sort of output.

Instead, it should be all right for us to say, "I kept my family alive today," and consider that a perfectly productive day. Or better yet, "I spent my whole day on the couch," and still feel like an accomplished, worthy human being. Some days that may be what we need to do, and we must trust that the benefits will seep into other days.

We Learned from Other Cultures

Countries around the world have a lot to teach us about living the good life. Despite the fact that I consider niksen to be much better for us than hygge and mindfulness, I'm glad all these wellness trends exist. Thanks to this variety, depending on your personal circumstances and characteristics, you can pick and choose the right one for you.

The Dutch know how to enjoy life, whether cycling through the dunes or the countryside or eating deep-fried snacks in a *gezellig* café. They can also teach us the importance of normalcy, which they say is crazy enough. In the spirit of keeping things normal, it would be a very Dutch

(195)

conclusion to say that niksen is great, but it's important not to overdo it. We need to be out and about too, not just at home niksening around, no matter how much I would love to do just that. We need friends and family and our colleagues and bosses.

At the same time, the desire to be free of work and responsibilities and take a little break every now and then is universal, no matter where we're from or where we live. In fact, I would even go so far as to say that it is the desire for niksen that connects us. Some of us call it niksen, while others go for *dolce far niente* or letting out your inner *Schweinehund* (pig dog) or even sweet, sweet nothing.

It takes some guts — or maybe even what the Jews call *chutzpah,* which means "audacity" or "extreme confidence" in Yiddish — to do nothing with abandon and without shame.

I think it's very important that we not shame others for the way they choose to spend their time. "There is value in differences, in knowing that people somewhere else lived differently and it worked for them. You could get little ideas or notions of what's possible," Irina Dumitrescu, the medieval researcher, says.

In my native Poland, we have the *jakos to bedzie* philosophy. This translates to "somehow it will be," and is the perfect phrase for tough times. "Happiness Polish style is getting out of your comfort zone. It's doing something that doesn't seem to make sense simply for the sake

of going against the tide. It's striving for change," To-
masz Lis, one of the coauthors of a book on the topic,
tells me. It's the kind of attitude we need to embrace
niksen.

We Could Fight Climate Change

There are other pressing issues to worry about too. The
last few summers have been the hottest so far, and many
scientists predict the future will be hotter still. The EU
has declared a climate crisis and is urging its members to
cut greenhouse emissions to zero by 2050. We may have
already tipped beyond the point of no return: polar ice
caps are melting; coral reefs are disappearing; the Amazon
rainforest experiences severe droughts; and, in countries
such as Sweden, Russia, Australia, and the US, dangerous
wildfires rage.

The Netherlands is situated largely below sea level, so
rising water levels are an imminent threat, and the question of climate change is even more pressing. "The year
2100, 2400, or 4000 AD could be a possible best-before
date for the Netherlands," writes Peter Kuipers Munneke
in an op-ed for the website of Utrecht University. As he
puts it, the question of the country disappearing is a matter of "when," and not "if." Dikes all over the country are
being fortified and raised, and there is promising technology being developed around floating houses. Innovators
are looking into working with water instead of against it,
but will this be enough?

(197)

We need smart decisions to deal with this crisis, and we need them now. While wellness trends from around the world do very little to help, focusing largely on the individual or just the home instead of preparing for what's coming, I believe niksen can offer us something new. We can't meditate the climate crisis away; we can't hygge in our homes while marginalized groups down the street are threatened. But we can niks for a short while and allow ourselves and our brains to recharge to come up with smarter solutions. And then we can get to work.

What's more, niksen is not a threat to the environment. We have brought climate change upon ourselves because we consume too much, waste too much, and do too much. When we do niks, there's none of that. A BBC article recently defended shorter workweeks, not because we are overworked, but in defense of the climate, killing two birds with one stone, so to speak.

It's time for us to bring this endless economic ambition to a halt. Constant economic growth requires we work harder and harder, but to what end? Even if the economy were to grow infinitely, can we be expected to always do more, buy and consume more, and tax the environment more?

(198)

The Solution? De-growth. Niks.

We Could Look for Contentment
Instead of Happiness

We all want to be happy — it's human nature. While studying niksen I spoke to many experts and researchers on happiness, and I realized that it is best seen not as a goal but more as a side effect of a well-lived life. I also found that it can mean such different things to different people. There simply isn't one way to feel happy or to become happy.

Many people get caught up in an almost reckless and stressful pursuit of happiness. I recommend that instead we strive toward something the Dutch do very well: contentment. They are happy, but not abundantly or extraordinarily so. Their happiness is generally more subdued, quieter. In fact, it's contentment that comes from them having ample free time, feeling like appreciated members of a community, and knowing they have a stable support network to fall back on should disaster strike, for instance in the form of sickness or unemployment.

In some cultures, the pursuit of happiness seems less pronounced, and it might even be perfectly fine to look quite miserable and not smile. Take the Polish, for instance, whose all-time favorite pastime is complaining, as described in *Jakos to bedzie: Szczescie po polsku,* by Daniel Lis. Polish people consider whining a way to bond with others, and so it brings about feelings of contentment.

Niksen gives us time to reflect, tune out, and think a little about what we like and don't like doing with our time. Niksen gives our lives meaning because it prioritizes what's important to us and encourages us to decide how we want to participate in society.

We Could Create Supportive Communities, Governments, and Neighborhoods

A Gallup poll from 2017 showed that many people in the US saw what they called "Big Government" as a threat. But policies that support parents, allow people to take time off, and protect the weakest members of society are more than a matter of common sense. These policies also boost happiness and well-being. A study by the Council of Contemporary Families found that in countries where parents were the most supported, the happiness gap between parents and non-parents was the smallest. The country where that gap was the highest? The US.

As family historian Stephanie Coontz argues in *The Way We Never Were,* "Children do best in societies where child-rearing is considered too important to be left entirely to parents." No wonder the Dutch have the world's happiest children: their parents have a lot of support from the government, daycare facilities, and extended family.

"When you take an idea that is very individual and apply it to a social context, I think that could be a very nice route," says Tony Crabbe, referring to niksen.

We need what Nakita Valerio, a Canada-based writer

and community organizer, calls "community care," which Valerio describes in an article as "people committed to leveraging their privilege to be there for one another in various ways." And the same can be said about self-care: it is too important to be left entirely to the individual. We need to do better as a society and demand our governments feel invested in our well-being.

A More Peaceful World Thanks to Niksen?

As the world changes, the Netherlands changes too. And not all change is for the better. "Social networks are important but less important than they used to be. Politics have become less socially supportive. There have been cuts, and not enough money is being spent on health care and social security," summarizes Carolien Hamming.

This causes heightened stress levels for the Dutch. "This is especially visible in statistics on burnout, for instance. And we also see changes among students: They're stressed because schools these days have higher expectations of them," Hamming continues.

Traditional Dutch characteristics such as the love of normalcy are changing too. These days, some of the Dutch want to be exceptional, which is new. "The ambition to be excellent is growing. We are a small country, and everyone knows us, we want to be known as heroes," says Catharina Haverkamp. But she adds: "There are voices telling us to be careful with that. It's better for children to feel they don't need to excel. It's better to know how to be yourself and know what your talents are, what you are good at, and focus on that. We don't all have to be heroes."

"That's why I like niksen," Haverkamp tells me. "We need to put niksen on our schedules. We need time to do nothing, to just absorb . . . to stop running, for more silence." Niksen, according to Haverkamp, can help us deal with this rapidly changing world and give us time to reflect on new ways to live and to be together and connect.

Kari Leibowitz agrees. "I think you need both the individual mind-set, but you also need institutional change. Individuals shape the culture and culture shapes individuals," she says. The way forward is through communities and, as Tony Crabbe calls them, niksen neighborhoods, where it's acceptable to do niks, take a break, and just sit in the sun for a while.

So while I'm anxious about the future, I also see change is underway. I see many people embracing a slower lifestyle and time for reflection. I see people refusing to be busy and trying to find time for their favorite activities or niksen. I see such a huge interest in niksen. And this gives me hope.

Sweet, Sweet Nothing

The day I typed the period after the last word in this book, I took a moment to take in the enormity of what I had just done. I had written a book. Wasn't that something? I gazed at the computer for a few more seconds and added a couple of final edits before sending this last chapter to my editor. And then I just gazed at the computer a little longer, for no reason whatsoever.

I noticed in my throat a familiar scratch, the end of a cold that had been with me for the last ten days. I was just starting to feel better. Or maybe this was the beginning of a new cold, you can just never tell with Dutch weather.

Then, just like any other Thursday, I went to my Dutch class and sped to the store to buy groceries for dinner. I got home just in time to see the school bus pull into our driveway. I made the children snacks and tried to keep them occupied until it was time to make dinner. I was going to make my daughter's favorite fried rice recipe.

But before cooking, I rolled out the croissant dough that had been sitting in my fridge waiting for me. Baking croissants is very time-consuming business. You have to pay attention to so many details, from the exact temperature of the butter to the exact number of times you have folded the dough, to get the delicious flaky layers so typical of this pastry. A lot can go wrong, so you have to be vigilant. In fact, when I make croissants, pretty much everything goes wrong.

(203)

But baking croissants also allows for plenty of niksen time while the dough is rising or resting or while the butter is cooling. In my busy life, croissants give me the chance to slow down, forcing me now and then to do nothing.

After dinner, I cleaned up and somehow got the kids into their pajamas. Once I put them to bed, and before my husband came home, I sat down on our new, shiny brown couch and covered myself with a blanket. Then I did nothing at all, and it was delicious.

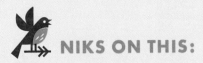

NIKS ON THIS:

- What do you think of the niksen philosophy?

- Do you think it can help us deal with an increasingly uncertain, globalized, and overwhelming world?

- What parts of the book seemed the most helpful to you?

(205)

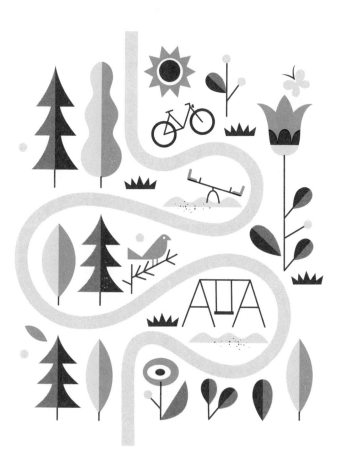

The Nikseneers' Manifesto

Who Are We?

We are the Nikseneers. Our name stems from *niksen,* which is a Dutch word for "doing nothing." Niksen is a Dutch lifestyle philosophy that refers to doing nothing without a purpose. That is, we don't do nothing to become calmer, better human beings. We do it just because.

To do niks does not mean to work, to perform emotional labor, or to be mindful. Nor is it selfish, lazy, or boring. On the contrary, niksen can be a service to the community. And it's not browsing Facebook, watching Netflix, or checking your email. You might call those things nothing, but in reality, they are not.

The desire to do nothing has been around forever and is part of every culture in the world. Think of the British Idler movement, the Italian notion of *dolce far niente,* or the Chinese philosophy of *wu wei.* It is absolutely normal to want to do nothing.

We, the Nikseneers, are done with wellness trends that tell us we should do more, buy more, or be better. We're fine just the way we are, and we're owning it.

What Do We Believe?

We believe that doing nothing can ultimately make us more productive. By taking breaks during our daily work, we can become better employees, avoid burnout, and work more carefully and deliberately.

We believe that niksen can make us more creative by giving us time to come up with ideas that are truly new and original instead of regurgitating old ones. Niksen gives time for our thoughts to interact, which results in insights that we may not have come up with otherwise.

And we believe that niksen makes us better decision makers by giving our unconscious brains time to go over all the possible options and choose the best one.

We believe that everyone deserves a break from work, from family, or from working out without being told that we are not enough or being judged for what we do (or don't do).

What Do We Want?

We want less busyness and more free time for our interests, hobbies, and passions. We want more time to do niks.

Niksen shouldn't be only the individual's responsibility. We want supportive countries, cities, societies, and neighborhoods. We want a more equal division of labor so that everyone can get their niksen time. We want recognition for the various invisible, unnoticed, and undervalued forms of labor that are often performed by the most vulnerable.

We want the right to play, fool around, experiment, and try out new things. And then after that is done, we want to be able to sit and contemplate the patterns on our rugs and slowly figure out what to do next. We want society to become more open toward niksen and not judge us when we do niks.

We want to redefine productivity so that our worth is not connected to how many hours we work each week or how much we produce.

We want to make the world more niksen friendly, and that starts with us.

Join us in our Facebook group, The Nikseneers: The People Who Love Doing Nothing!

Quick Niksen Tips

At Work

- Use a part of your work break for niksen. Stare at your computer, take in the view from your office, close your eyes.
- After you order your lunch, while you wait for it to be prepared, don't check your phone but instead sit down and do nothing for a while.
- When you notice that you can't focus, step away from the computer and engage in some niksen.
- When commuting to and from work by train, spend a few minutes just doing nothing for a change. Resist the urge to browse Facebook and read emails.
- If you're stuck in traffic, don't give in to road rage. Instead: breathe . . . and enjoy doing nothing.
- If possible, find a quiet room or area for niksen.
- When you've just arrived for work, don't rush into your day. Try to switch from home mode to work

mode by sitting down for a few minutes and doing nothing.

- Do the same after you've finished work and are ready to go home.
- You can niksen in between tasks to make the transition smoother.
- Go to meetings only when your presence is required; instead, use that freed-up time to do nothing.

At Home

- Organize your home so that it becomes niksen friendly. Comfy chairs, sofas, and reading nooks are great ways to help you ease into niksen time.
- When you're not working or doing chores, try to relax by sitting down and doing nothing, even if it's just for a few minutes before you have to go and take care of the next thing.
- If you work from home, remember that you're also entitled to work breaks and can use chunks of that time for niksen.
- Remember that doing chores, performing emotional labor, and raising children are work and you should therefore feel entitled to take breaks from those things too.
- Mark the end of every chore by niksening for a few minutes.
- When reading a book, put it away for a while and

spend a couple of minutes doing nothing (or maybe thinking about what the characters are doing).

- When you find yourself mindlessly browsing Facebook, stop and do niks.
- When you're tired after a long day at work or with the children (or both) but you don't want to go to bed yet, niks away.
- When you're in bed but can't fall asleep, get up and make yourself some chamomile tea and niks with it. Or stay in bed and do nothing for a while.

Out in Public

- When you go somewhere via public transportation, don't grab your phone but instead spend a few minutes doing nothing.
- Same if you're stuck in traffic.
- Nature, such as the beach, the park, the forest, or the mountains, is a perfect place for niksen.
- If you have to wait for the bus, think of that as niksen time.
- Same if you're waiting for your doctor's appointment.
- Or any appointment, really.
- When your children are busy with activities that don't require your constant attention, use that time to do nothing.
- While at the playground with your kids, you can

switch off for a while instead of scrolling through your social media. (No judgment here, we've all done it.)

- When you're in a café or restaurant waiting for your date or friend to arrive, do nothing for a few minutes.
- When you're at the theater or cinema, before the performance or movie starts, take a while to mentally prepare yourself for the entertainment ahead by . . . doing nothing.

Niksen Tips from the Dutch

1. Be direct.

Dutch directness can be perplexing to people from other cultures where social norms of politeness and manners prevent direct, honest comments from ever being said. And so the Dutch often come across as rude. But from the Dutch perspective, there is nothing rude about directness at all. It's simply communication.

I must admit that I initially found Dutch directness upsetting. But I have learned to appreciate it, and I can see it has advantages. It allows parties to clear the air very quickly. The Dutch cut through the fluff and give you facts — or their opinion. If you get directness right, it can be very, very effective, not to mention efficient. So, if you're niksening, don't be afraid to talk about it openly.

2. Be tolerant of other people's niksen time.

A typical trait of the Dutch is the so-called *verzuiling,* or "pillarization," which can be described as "to each their own" or "live and let live." What this means is that while everyone is expected to contribute to society, just about all lifestyle choices are either openly accepted or at least tolerated. In addition, all groups of society have the right to stand up and voice their opinions. Decisions are made by consensus.

As a result, even if some people in the Netherlands are opposed to niksen, nikseneers will be able to get their niksen time without intolerance from others.

3. Create a niksen-friendly environment.
In the Netherlands, nature is taken care of and protected. Your environment affects the way you feel, and maybe this is one of the reasons the Dutch are happy. So why not learn from that and make your house and office niksen friendly? Decorate with comfortable couches and create niksen nooks for yourself. Bring in calm-inducing colors such as greens and blues. Position your furniture facing a fireplace or a window, not the TV. Keep your devices where they are available to you should you need them, but out of sight, so you won't be tempted to get online all the time.

Wherever you live, you'll find niksen-friendly benches in parks, on building roofs, on balconies, or in natural environments such as woods, beaches, or dunes. Go out and find a few favorite spots to niksen in.

4. Put niksen on the agenda.
The Dutch don't do anything without consulting their schedules first. This might be hard for people who are

more spontaneous with their social lives, but that's how the Dutch make sure there is time for everything that a good life comprises: work, friendships, family, hobbies, sports, and relaxation. I think this is great, because if they can be organized about scheduling appointments, they can be organized about carving out niksen time too. Think about it: You already use your agenda to schedule everything else, so why not schedule some niksen time too? It is just as important for your mental and physical health as seeing your doctor.

5. Look for niksen pockets during your day.
One of the reasons some of the Dutch are skeptical about niksen is because they are calling it something else, such as cycling, going to the beach, or hanging out with friends. But there are moments, for example after swimming in the North Sea on a sunny day, when the Dutch just lie down (on their towels on the sand) and really do niks.

You can do the same, and you don't even need a beach. If you pay attention, you'll find plenty of niksen moments to enjoy: while you're waiting for the doctor to see you or while you're waiting for a bus, for instance. I call these moments "niksen pockets," and all you have to do to start enjoying that niksen time is keep an eye open for them.

6. Just be normal.
In the Netherlands, extreme outbursts of emotion are seen as weird or even insincere or fake. A typical saying in this country is *doe maar gewoon, dan ben je al gek genoeg,*

or in English, "just be normal, that's crazy enough." In the Netherlands, it's not accepted to complain or brag about working all the time. It's not considered nice to boast about your accomplishments or to differentiate yourself from others. Don't try to be a superhero. Just be normal.

And remember, it's absolutely natural to want to do nothing. In fact, it's normal.

7. Be critical.

The Dutch are critical thinkers, and they are unlikely to just accept any new trend that they encounter. It's good to be cautious of new wellness trends that promise to make you fit, healthy, and perfect, because chances are, they won't.

At the same time, it's perfectly acceptable for a Dutch person to change their point of view the moment new information becomes available. So, do like the Dutch: try niksen and see if it works for you. If not, try it again in a different setting and see what happens. And if that doesn't work either, try something else completely. No harm done.

Acknowledgments

I expected writing this book to be hard work, and it was. But I didn't think it would be so much fun. This is, for the biggest part, thanks to my fabulous editor, Hedi de Vree. When you told me to "have fun" writing this book, I didn't believe you. But you were right all along. Your witty and thoughtful edits were right to the point and made this book so much better.

Working with Hedi and others at Kosmos Uitgevers was every writer's dream. Writing a book can be a lonely experience, so it's really important to have someone holding your hand and providing you with both gentle guidance and tough deadlines.

Carrie Ballard, your watchful eyes have caught every typo, mistake, and inconsistency.

Julia Foldenyi, Irina Formichev, and everyone at Shared Stories, it was your dedication to the book and your belief in its message that made it possible for *Niksen* to appear in so many languages.

Deb Brody and Emma Peters, at Houghton Mifflin

Harcourt, thank you for your interest in niksen. Your help and support and kind edits were instrumental in bringing this book to a North American audience. At HMH, I also want to thank Rebecca Springer for asking all the right questions and finding all the right words and Bridget Nocera for her help and advice on effective book marketing. Thanks also to art director Martha Kennedy, interior designer Chrissy Kurpeski, and illustrator Tracy Walker.

Theresa Fisher, by accepting my quirky story on doing literally nothing for publication on *Woolly Magazine,* you have given the niksen philosophy a perfect home and started something I could never have foreseen.

Tim Herrera, when you emailed me back after rejecting my niksen idea for the *New York Times* Smarter Living section and wrote these epic words, "Maybe we could revisit this?" you changed my life. You'll always have my gratitude.

Michele Hutchison and Marei Pittner, thank you for your valuable advice on publishing and translation rights. I learned a lot from talking to you when it came to navigating the confusing world of traditional publishing!

I'm very lucky to have a team of clever, dedicated women to help with social media. To Hanna Cheda, my trusted virtual assistant, for holding down the fort while I was writing this book and to Pinar Tarhan for your help running The Nikseneers: thank you.

Thank you to my husband, Nikolai, without whom I'd be totally and utterly lost — in both the metaphorical and literal sense of the word.

My children were on their best behavior while I wrote this book and also contributed wise insights and ideas. Thank you for "Mama, you should write about this." And when they found out that my namesake and fellow countrywoman Olga Tokarczuk was awarded the Nobel Prize in Literature in 2019, they said, "That means you'll be next!" Thank you for believing in me.

Thank you also to my parents, Ewa and Aleksy Bartnik, for supporting me and being proud of me; my brother, Witek Bartnik, for repairing my printer when I needed it most; my sister-in-law Gosia Cwil, for the many great discussions we had about work and having time off; and my in-laws, Eva and Michael Mecking, for the many interesting discussions we had about niksen and for their support and encouragement when I told them about the book.

Thank you also to the people of the Netherlands, for giving me a home, and to the ladies at the Dutch daycare in Delft, who saved my sanity, and probably my life too. Marjan Simons, your passion for the Dutch language is contagious. *Hartelijk bedankt* for passing it on to me.

To everyone on the internet, thanks for helping me decide whether my niksen-friendly couch (which is also brown, new, and shiny) was a shiny, new, brown couch or a new shiny brown couch. I still have little clarity in this matter. But on that day, you made my day when I needed it most.

My favorite Facebook groups: The Binders, Multicultural Kid Blogs, BLUNTmoms, and, of course, The Nikseneers — thank you!!

Bibliography

INTRODUCTION: Oh No, Not Another Wellness Trend!

Altman, Anna. "The Year of Hygge, the Danish Obsession with Getting Cozy." *The New Yorker,* December 18, 2016. https://www.newyorker.com/culture/culture-desk/the-year-of-hygge-the-danish-obsession-with-getting-cozy.

Cederström, Carl, and André Spicer. *The Wellness Syndrome.* Polity, 2015.

Corliss, Julie. "Mindfulness Meditation May Ease Anxiety, Mental Stress." *Harvard Health Publishing,* January 8, 2014. https://www.health.harvard.edu/blog/mindfulness-meditation-may-ease-anxiety-mental-stress-201401086967.

Dolan, Paul. *Happy Ever After: Escaping the Myth of the Perfect Life.* Allen Lane, 2019.

Ehrenreich, Barbara. *Natural Causes: An Epidemic of Wellness, the Certainty of Dying, and Killing Ourselves to Live Longer.* Twelve, 2019.

Gallup 2019. "Global Emotions Report." https://www.gallup.com/analytics/248906/gallup-global-emotions-report-2019.aspx.

"German Word of the Day: *Die Gemütlichkeit.*" *The Local,* September 27, 2018. https://www.thelocal.de/20180927/die-gemuetlichkeit.

"Half of Brits Feel 'Time Poor' and Majority Are Too Stressed to Have

Fun." *Mirror,* July 13, 2017. https://www.mirror.co.uk/news
/uk-news/half-brits-feel-time-poor-10791478.

Knoll, Jessica. "Smash the Wellness Industry." *New York Times,* June
8, 2019. https://www.nytimes.com/2019/06/08/opinion/sunday/
women-dieting-wellness.html.

Kondo, Marie. *The Life-Changing Magic of Tidying Up: A Simple, Effective Way to Banish Clutter Forever.* Vermilion, 2014.

Mecking, Olga. "The Case for Doing Nothing." *New York Times,* April
29, 2019. https://www.nytimes.com/2019/04/29/smarter-living
/the-case-for-doing-nothing.html.

"Mental Health Statistics: Stress." Mental Health Foundation. https://
www.mentalhealth.org.uk/statistics/mental-health-statistics-stress.

Oppong, Thomas. "Ikigai: The Japanese Secret to a Long and Happy
Life Might Just Help You Live a More Fulfilling Life." Thrive Global,
Medium, January 10, 2018. https://medium.com/thrive-global
/ikigai-the-japanese-secret-to-a-long-and-happy-life-might-just
-help-you-live-a-more-fulfilling-9871d01992b7.

Taylor, Daron. "The 'Hygge' Trend Took America by Storm. Just Don't
Try to Translate It." *Washington Post,* March 22, 2018. https://www
.washingtonpost.com/news/worldviews/wp/2018/03/22/the
-hygge-trend-took-america-by-storm-just-dont-try-to-translate-it.

Thomson, Lizzie. "What You Need to Know About the Korean Wellness Concept 'Nunchi.'" *Metro,* August 19, 2019. https://metro.
co.uk/2019/08/19/what-you-need-to-know-about-the-korean
-wellness-concept-nunchi-10591394.

Twenge, Jean M. "Have Smartphones Destroyed a Generation?" *The
Atlantic,* September 2017. https://www.theatlantic.com/magazine
/archive/2017/09/has-the-smartphone-destroyed-a-generation
/534198.

——. "Why So Many People Are Stressed and Depressed." *Psychology
Today,* February 10, 2014. https://www.psychologytoday.com
/us/blog/our-changing-culture/201410/why-so-many-people
-are-stressed-and-depressed.

Verhoeven, Gebke. "Niksen Is the New Mindfulness." *Gezond Nu,*

August 24, 2017. https://gezondnu.nl/dossiers/psyche/stress
/niksen-het-nieuwe-mindfulness.

Winant, Gabriel. "Mind Control: Barbara Ehrenreich's Radical Critique
of Wellness and Self-Improvement." *New Republic,* May 23, 2018.
https://newrepublic.com/article/148296/barbara-ehrenreich
-radical-critique-wellness-culture.

Yankovich, Gyan, "A Beginner's Guide to Swedish Death Cleaning."
Buzzfeed, April 1, 2018. https://www.buzzfeed.com/gyanyankovich
/what-is-swedish-death-cleaning.

"Zen Buddhism." BBC. http://www.bbc.co.uk/religion/religions
/buddhism/subdivisions/zen_1.shtml.

CHAPTER 1: What Is Niksen?

Bradt, Steve, "Wandering Mind Not a Happy Mind." November
11, 2010. *Harvard Gazette.* https://news.harvard.edu/gazette/
story/2010/11/wandering-mind-not-a-happy-mind.

De Bres, Elise. "The Power of *Niksen* and *Lantefanteren*." Boek/Coach,
January 26, 2018. https://boekcoach.nl/the-power-niksen-and
-lantefanteren.

Demers, Dawn. "More Than Bubble Baths: The Real Definition of
Self-Care." Thrive Global, September 24, 2019. https://thriveglobal
.com/stories/more-than-bubble-baths-the-real-definition-of-self
-care.

Dodgen-Magee, Doreen. *Deviced!: Balancing Life and Technology in
a Digital World.* Rowman & Littlefield Publishers, 2018.

Eastwood, John E., et al. "The Unengaged Mind: Defining Boredom in
Terms of Attention." *Perspectives on Psychological Science,*
September 5, 2015. https://journals.sagepub.com/doi/abs
/10.1177/1745691612456044.

Frank, Priscilla. "'Boring Self-Care' Drawings Celebrate Everyday
Mental Health Victories." *HuffPost,* May 15, 2015. https://www
.huffpost.com/entry/boring-self-care_n_5914dabae4b00f308cf
40a19.

Gottfried, Sophia. "Niksen Is the Dutch Lifestyle Concept of Doing Nothing—And You're About to See It Everywhere." *Time,* July 12, 2019. https://time.com/5622094/what-is-niksen.

Hartley, Gemma. *Fed Up: Emotional Labor, Women, and the Way Forward.* HarperOne, 2018.

"Innerer Schweinehund." Wictionary. https://en.wiktionary.org/wiki/innerer_Schweinehund.

"Luieren." Encyclo.nl. https://www.encyclo.nl/begrip/luieren.

The Nikseneers—People Who Love Doing Nothing. Facebook. https://www.facebook.com/groups/TheNikseneers.

Odell, Jenny. *How to Do Nothing: Resisting the Attention Economy.* Melville House, 2019.

"People Spend 'Half Their Waking Hours Daydreaming.'" BBC, November 12, 2010. https://www.bbc.com/news/health-11741350.

Renz, Katie. "How To Be Idle: An Interview with Tom Hodgkinson." *Mother Jones,* June 8, 2005. https://www.motherjones.com/media/2005/06/how-be-idle-interview-tom-hodgkinson.

Rubin, Gretchen. "Put the Word 'Meditation' Before a Boring Task, Competitive Parenting, and Ideas for Organizing Recipes." *Happier with Gretchen Rubin* Podcast 53. https://gretchenrubin.com/podcast-episode/parenting-happier-podcast-53.

Wiest, Brianna. "This Is What 'Self-Care' REALLY Means, Because It's Not All Salt Baths and Chocolate Cake." *Thought Catalog,* January 14, 2020. https://thoughtcatalog.com/brianna-wiest/2017/11/this-is-what-self-care-really-means-because-its-not-all-salt-baths-and-chocolate-cake.

CHAPTER 2: What If the Dutch Got It Right?

Acosta, Rina Mae, and Michele Hutchison. *The Happiest Kids in the World: How Dutch Parents Help Their Kids (and Themselves) by Doing Less.* The Experiment, April 4, 2017.

Adam, Hajo, et al. "How Living Abroad Helps You Develop a Clearer Sense of Self." *Harvard Business Review,* May 22, 2018. https://

hbr.org/2018/05/how-living-abroad-helps-you-develop-a-clearer
-sense-of-self.

Amos, Jonathan. "Dutch Men Revealed as World's Tallest." BBC,
July 26, 2016. https://www.bbc.com/news/science-environment
-36888541.

Balicki, Jan. *Amsterdamskie ABC.* Iskry, 1974.

Bandy, Lauren. "New Nutrition Data Shows Global Calorie Consumption." *Euromonitor,* February 2, 2015. https://blog.euromonitor.com
/new-nutrition-data-shows-global-calorie-consumption.

Barry, Ellen. "A Peculiarly Dutch Summer Rite: Children Let Loose in
the Night Woods." *New York Times,* July 21, 2019. https://www
.nytimes.com/2019/07/21/world/europe/netherlands-dropping
-children.html.

Becker, Sascha O., and Ludger Woessmann. "Economics Helps Explain
Why Suicide Is More Common Among Protestants." *Aeon,* January
14, 2019. https://aeon.co/ideas/economics-helps-explain-why
-suicide-is-more-common-among-protestants.

"Best in Travel 2020 Top Countries." Lonely Planet. https://www
.lonelyplanet.com/best-in-travel/countries.

Billinghurst, Stuart. "Dutch Circle Party Guide — How to Survive a
Dutch Birthday." *Invading Holland,* October 5, 2018. https://www
.invadingholland.com/guides-to-holland/the-dutch-circle-party
-guide.

Boffey, Daniel. "Dutch Government Ditches Holland to Rebrand as the
Netherlands." *Guardian,* October 4, 2019. https://www.theguardian
.com/world/2019/oct/04/holland-the-netherlands-dutch
-government-rebrand.

Burnett, Dean. "Crack and Cheese: Do Pleasurable Things Really Affect Your Brain Like Drugs?" *Guardian,* February 13, 2018. https://
www.theguardian.com/science/brain-flapping/2018/feb/13/crack
-and-cheese-do-pleasurable-things-really-affect-your-brain
-like-drugs.

Coates, Ben. *Why the Dutch Are Different: A Journey into the Hidden
Heart of the Netherlands.* Nicholas Brealey, 2017.

"Country Report: The Netherlands." Hofstede Insights. https://www
.hofstede-insights.com/country/the-netherlands.

Daly, Mary C., et al. "Dark Contrasts: The Paradox of High Rates of
Suicide in Happy Places." *Journal of Economic Behavior & Organization,* December 2011. https://www.researchgate.net/
publication/228462399_Dark_Contrasts_The_Paradox_of_
High_Rates_of_Suicide_in_Happy_Places.

de Bruin, Ellen. *Dutch Women Don't Get Depressed.* Contact, 2007.

Dillon, Connor. "Obese? Not Us! Why the Netherlands Is Becoming
the Skinniest EU Country." *Deutsche Welle,* June 9, 2015. https://
www.dw.com/en/obese-not-us-why-the-netherlands-is
-becoming-the-skinniest-eu-country/a-18503808.

Ducharme, Jamie. "Trying to Be Happy Is Making You Miserable.
Here's Why." *Time,* August 10, 2018. https://time.com/5356657
/trying-to-be-happy.

Epstein, David. *Range: Why Generalists Triumph in a Specialized
World.* Riverhead Books, 2019.

Falk, John H., and John D. Balling. "Evolutionary Influence on Human
Landscape Preference." *Environment and Behavior,* August 7, 2009.
https://www.researchgate.net/publication/249624620_Evolution
ary_Influence_on_Human_Landscape_Preference.

Ferrari, Alize J., et al. "Burden of Depressive Disorders by Country,
Sex, Age, and Year: Findings from the Global Burden of
Disease Study 2010." *PLOS Medicine,* November 5, 2013. https://
journals.plos.org/plosmedicine/article?id=10.1371/journal
.pmed.1001547.

Fischer, Jake. "NBA Players Have a New Favorite Snack: Energy-Boost-
ing Stroopwafels." *Washington Post,* December 4, 2019.
https://www.washingtonpost.com/sports/2019/12/05/nba-waffles
-stroopwafel-robert-covington-honeystinger.

Guiliano, Mireille. *French Women Don't Get Fat. The Secret of Eating
for Pleasure.* Vintage, 2007.

Harkness, Sara, and Charles M. Super. "Themes and Variations: Parental Ethnotheories in Western Cultures." In K. H. Rubin and O. B.

Chung (eds.), *Parental Beliefs, Parenting, and Child Development in Cross-Cultural Perspective.* Psychology Press, 2006.

Jacobs Hendel, Hilary. "Ignoring Your Emotions Is Bad for Your Health. Here's What to Do About It." *Time,* February 27, 2018. https://time.com/5163576/ignoring-your-emotions-bad-for-your-health.

Lauletta, Tyler. "Megan Rapinoe Proved All of Her Haters Wrong with One of the Most Brilliant Performances in World Cup History." *Business Insider,* July 9, 2019. https://www.businessinsider.nl/megan-rapinoe-trump-womens-world-cup-2019-7?international=true&r=US.

Mecking, Olga. "Saving the Dynamic Ecosystems of the Dutch Dunes." *Deutsche Welle,* September 29, 2019. https://www.dw.com/en/saving-the-dynamic-ecosystems-of-the-dutch-dunes/a-50471813.

M. S. "Who's Watching?" *Economist,* February 12, 2014. https://www.economist.com/charlemagne/2014/02/12/whos-watching.

Oka, Noriyuki, and Sophia Ankel. "Why You Should Opt for the Dutch De-Stressing Method 'Niksen' over 'Hygge,' According to a Health Expert." *Business Insider,* January 1, 2020. https://www.insider.com/niksen-replacing-hygge-as-the-best-method-de-stressing-method-2019-11.

"Oxfam Food Index." Oxfam of America. January 14, 2013. https://s3.amazonaws.com/oxfam-us/www/static/media/files/Good_Enough_To_Eat_Media_brief_FINAL.pdf.

"Parental Leave." The Newbie Guide to Sweden. https://www.thenewbieguide.se/just-arrived/register-for-welfare/parental-leave.

Pellman Rowland, Michael. "This Is Your Brain On Cheese." *Forbes,* June 26, 2017. https://www.forbes.com/sites/michaelpellmanrowland/2017/06/26/cheese-addiction/#37cf26a13583.

Pieters, Janene. "US Stunned by 'Peculiarly Dutch' Rite of 'Dropping.'" *Netherlands Times,* July 22, 2019. https://nltimes.nl/2019/07/22/us-stunned-peculiarly-dutch-rite-dropping.

Oishi, Shigehiro, et al. "Personality and Geography: Introverts Prefer Mountains." *Journal of Research in Personality,* July 27, 2015. https://

www.researchgate.net/publication/279754847_Personality_and
_Geography_Introverts_Prefer_Mountains.

Ward, Claire. "How Dutch Women Got to Be the Happiest in the
World." *Maclean's,* August 19, 2011. https://www.macleans.ca/news
/world/the-feminismhappiness-axis.

Woolcot, Simon. "How to Make Friends with the Dutch." *Amsterdam
Shallow Man,* September 2013. https://amsterdamshallowman.
com/2013/09/how-to-make-friends-with-the-dutch.html.

"World Happiness Report 2019." World Happiness Report, March 20,
2019. https://worldhappiness.report/ed/2019.

CHAPTER 3: Why Is Niksen So Hard?

Bates, Sofie. "A Decade of Data Reveals That Heavy Multitaskers Have
Reduced Memory, Stanford Psychologist Says." *Stanford News,* October 25, 2018. https://news.stanford.edu/2018/10/25/decade-data
-reveals-heavy-multitaskers-reduced-memory-psychologist-says.

Cain Miller, Claire. "Women Did Everything Right. Then Work Got
'Greedy.'" *New York Times,* April 26, 2019. https://www.nytimes
.com/2019/04/26/upshot/women-long-hours-greedy-professions
.html.

Cook, Chris. "Why Are Steiner Schools So Controversial?" BBC News,
August 4, 2014. https://www.bbc.com/news/education-28646118.

Crabbe, Tony. *Busy: How to Thrive in a World of Too Much.* Grand
Central Publishing, 2015.

Dolan, Paul. *Happy Ever After: Escaping the Myth of the Perfect Life.* Allen Lane, 2019.

Dumitrescu, Irina. "'Bio-Nazis' Go Green in Germany." *Politico,* July 13,
2018. https://www.politico.eu/article/germany-bio-nazis-go
-green-natural-farming-right-wing-extremism.

Ehrenreich, Barbara. *Bright-sided: How Positive Thinking Is Undermin-
ing America.* Henry Holt and Company, 2009.

Eschner, Kat. "A Little History of American Kindergartens." *Smithson-*

ian Magazine, May 16, 2017. https://www.smithsonianmag.com
/smart-news/little-history-american-kindergartens-180963263.

Fleming, Peter. "Do You Work More Than 39 Hours a Week? Your Job
Could Be Killing You." *Guardian,* January 15, 2018. https://www
.theguardian.com/lifeandstyle/2018/jan/15/is-28-hours-ideal
-working-week-for-healthy-life.

Frazer, John. "How the Gig Economy Is Reshaping Careers for the Next
Generation." *Forbes,* February 15, 2019. https://www.forbes.com
/sites/johnfrazer1/2019/02/15/how-the-gig-economy-is-reshaping
-careers-for-the-next-generation.

Gabriele, Ludo. *Woke Daddy.* http://wokedaddy.com.

"Health & Wellness Industry Statistics 2019 [Latest Market Data &
Trends]." Wellness Creative Co., July 3, 2019. https://www
.wellnesscreatives.com/wellness-industry-statistics.

Ko, Youkyung. "Sebastian Kneipp and the Natural Cure Movement
of Germany: Between Naturalism and Modern Medicine." *Korean
Journal of Medical History* 25, no. 3 (2016): 557–590. https://doi
.org/10.13081/kjmh.2016.25.557

Kross, Ethan, et al. "Social Rejection Shares Somatosensory Represen-
tations with Physical Pain." *Proceedings of the National Academy of
Sciences of the United States of America* 108, no. 15 (2011):
6270–6275. https://doi.org/10.1073/pnas.1102693108.

Lieberman, Matthew D. *Social: Why Our Brains Are Wired to Connect.*
Crown, 2013.

MacEacheran, Mike. "How Switzerland Transformed Breakfast." BBC
Travel, August 14, 2017. http://www.bbc.com/travel/story/20170808
-how-switzerland-transformed-breakfast.

Marsh, Stefanie. "Gabrielle Deydier: What It's Like to Be Fat in France."
Guardian, September 10, 2017. https://www.theguardian.com
/society/2017/sep/10/gabrielle-deydier-fat-in-france-abuse
-grossophobia-book-women.

McMunn, Anne, et al. "Gender Divisions of Paid and Unpaid Work in
Contemporary UK Couples." *Work, Employment and Society,* July
25, 2019. https://doi.org/10.1177/0950017019862153.

More Muelle, Christina. "The History of Kindergarten: From

Germany to the United States." 2013. https://digitalcommons.fiu
.edu/cgi/viewcontent.cgi?referer=&httpsredir=1&article=1110&con
text=sferc.

Mullainathan, Sendhil, and Eldar Shafir. *Scarcity: Why Having Too Little Means So Much.* Times Books, 2013.

"Parents Now Spend Twice as Much Time with Their Children as 50
Years Ago." *Economist,* November 27, 2017. https://www.economist
.com/graphic-detail/2017/11/27/parents-now-spend-twice-as-much
-time-with-their-children-as-50-years-ago.

Pollen, Annebella. "Looking Back at Life Reform: Movements and
Methods for Turbulent Times." *Corrupted Files,* February 2018.
http://www.corruptedfiles.org.uk/portfolio/looking-back-at-life
-reform.

Sanbonmatsu, David M., et al. "Who Multi-Tasks and Why? Multi-
Tasking Ability, Perceived Multi-Tasking Ability, Impulsivity,
and Sensation Seeking." *PLOS ONE,* January 23, 2013. https://doi
.org/10.1371/journal.pone.0054402.

Savage, Maddy. "The 'Paradox' of Working in the World's Most Equal
Countries." BBC Worklife, September 4, 2019. https://www.bbc
.com/worklife/article/20190831-the-paradox-of-working-in-the
-worlds-most-equal-countries.

Schaffer, Amanda. "How the Brain Seeks Pleasure and Avoids Pain."
MIT Technology Review, June 27, 2017. https://www.technology
review.com/s/608000/how-the-brain-seeks-pleasure-and-avoids
-pain.

Schröder, Christian. "Sich frei machen, um frei zu leben: Geschichte
der Lebensreformbewegung." *Der Tagesspiegel,* June 26, 2017.
https://www.tagesspiegel.de/gesellschaft/geschichteder
-lebensreformbewegung-nicht-die-welt-sondern-das-ich-soll
-verbessert-werden/19971278-4.html.

Scott, Elizabeth. "How to Deal with FOMO in Your Life." *Verywell
Mind,* November 26, 2019. https://www.verywellmind.com/how
-to-cope-with-fomo-4174664.

Stillman, Jessica. "This Is the Ideal Number of Hours to Work a Day,
According to Decades of Science." *Inc.,* August 29, 2017. https://

www.inc.com/jessica-stillman/this-is-the-ideal-number-of-hours
-to-work-a-day-ac.html.

"Time Spent in Paid and Unpaid Work, by Sex." Organisation for
Economic Co-operation and Development. Data extracted on
January 25, 2020. https://stats.oecd.org/index.aspx?queryid
=54757

Vanderkam, Laura. *I Know How She Does It: How Successful Women
Make the Most of Their Time*. Portfolio, 2015.

Veblen, Thorstein. *The Theory of the Leisure Class: An Economic Study
of Institutions*. 1899. http://moglen.law.columbia.edu/LCS
/theoryleisureclass.pdf.

Wilson, Timothy D., et al. "The Mind in Its Own Place: The Difficul-
ties and Benefits of Thinking for Pleasure." *Advances in Experi-
mental Psychology* 60 (2019), 175–221. https://doi.org/10.1016/
bs.aesp.2019.05.001.

CHAPTER 4: Niksen Is Good for You. Yes, It Is.

Callard, Felicity, and Daniel S. Margulies. "What We Talk About When
We Talk About the Default Mode Network." *Frontiers in Human
Neuroscience*, August 25, 2014. https://www.ncbi.nlm.nih.gov/pmc/
articles/PMC4142807/pdf/fnhum-08-00619.pdf.

Cleese, John. "On Creativity in Management." https://www.youtube
.com/embed/Pb5oIIPO62g?start=60.

Dijksterhuis, Ap. "Think Different: The Merits of Unconscious
Thought in Preference Development and Decision Making." *Journal of Personality and Social Psychology*, November 2004. https://
doi.org/10.1037/0022-3514.87.5.586.

Hogarth, Robin M., et al. "The Two Settings of Kind and Wicked
Learning Environments." *Current Directions in Psychological Sciences*, October 1, 2015. https://doi.org/10.1177/0963721415591878.

Kahneman, Daniel, and Gary Klein. "Conditions for Intuitive Expertise: A Failure to Disagree." *American Psychologist*, October 2009.
https://doi.org/10.1037/a0016755.

————. *Thinking, Fast and Slow.* Farrar, Straus and Giroux, 2013.

Levitt, Steven D. "Heads or Tails: The Impact of a Coin Toss on Major Life Decisions and Subsequent Happiness." National Bureau of Economic Research, August 2016. https://www.nber.org/papers/w22487.pdf.

Mann, Sandi, and Rebekah Cadman. "Does Being Bored Make Us More Creative?" *Creativity Research Journal,* May 8, 2014. https://www.tandfonline.com/doi/abs/10.1080/10400419.2014.901073.

Mecking, Olga. "What Is a Gut Feeling, and Should You Trust It?" *Forge,* June 28, 2019. https://forge.medium.com/what-is-a-gut-feeling-and-should-you-trust-it-47f5245c9d4e.

Pozen, Robert C. *Extreme Productivity: Boost Your Results, Reduce Your Hours.* Harper Business, 2012.

Raichle, Marcus E., et al. "A Default Mode of Brain Function." *Proceedings of the National Academy of Sciences of the United States of America,* January 16, 2001. https://www.pnas.org/content/98/2/676.

CHAPTER 5: Niksening Up Your Life

Bailey, Chris. *The Productivity Project: Accomplishing More by Managing Your Time, Attention, and Energy.* Crown, 2016.

Belton, Teresa. "How Kids Can Benefit from Boredom." *The Conversation,* September 23, 2016. https://theconversation.com/how-kids-can-benefit-from-boredom-65596.

Bloem, Craig. "Why Successful People Wear the Same Thing Every Day." *Inc.,* February 20, 2018. https://www.inc.com/craig-bloem/this-1-unusual-habit-helped-make-mark-zuckerberg-steve-jobs-dr-dre-successful.html.

Fuda, Peter. "10 Reasons Effective Meetings Are So Important." *HuffPost,* December 6, 2017. https://www.huffpost.com/entry/10-reasons-why-effective_b_6130262.

Gilovich, Thomas, et al. "The Spotlight Effect in Social Judgment: An Egocentric Bias in Estimates of the Salience of One's Own Actions and Appearance." *Journal of Personality and Social Psychology,* June 6, 2000. https://doi.org/10.1037//0022-3514.78.2.211.

"Global Recommendations on Physical Activity for Health." World Health Organization, 2010. https://apps.who.int/iris/bitstream /handle/10665/44399/9789241599979_eng.pdf;jsessionid =830EFFAB847AFE421E0B7086CBA1D6D3?sequence=1.

Grose, Jessica. "Your Boss Should Take Full Parental Leave." *New York Times,* August 13, 2019. https://www.nytimes.com/2019/08/13 /parenting/parental-family-leave.html.

Johansson, Anna. "Why Meetings Are One of the Worst Business Rituals. Ever." *Entrepreneur Magazine,* April 8, 2015. https://www .entrepreneur.com/article/244499.

Jonat, Rachel. *The Joy of Doing Nothing: A Real-Life Guide to Stepping Back, Slowing Down, and Creating a Simpler, Joy-Filled Life.* Adams Media, 2017.

Martin, Wednesday. *Primates of Park Avenue: A Memoir.* Simon & Schuster, 2015.

Mecking, Olga. "The Sanity-Saving Approach to Housework." *O, The Oprah Magazine,* September 19, 2017. http://www.oprah.com /inspiration/how-to-handle-housework-efficiently.

The Nikseneers: The People Who Love Doing Nothing Facebook Group. https://www.facebook.com/groups/TheNikseneers.

Resnick, Brian. "Late Sleepers Are Tired of Being Discriminated Against. And Science Has Their Back." *Vox,* February 27, 2018. https://www.vox.com/science-and-health/2018/2/27/17058530.

Thaler, Richard H., and Cass R. Sunstein. *Nudge: Improving Decisions About Health, Wealth, and Happiness.* Revised and expanded edition. Penguin Books, 2009.

Tonelli, Lucia. "14 Calming Paint Colors That Will Change the Way You Live." *Elle Décor,* January 9, 2019. https://www.elledecor.com /design-decorate/color/a25781168/calming-colors.

Zetlin, Minda. "Do You Have a Not-to-Do List? Here's Why You Should." *Inc,* March 30, 2018. https://www.inc.com/minda-zetlin /got-a-to-do-list-great-a-not-to-do-list-is-even-more-important .html.

Chapter 6: When Niksen Doesn't Work

Avent, Ryan. "Why Do We Work So Hard?" *Economist,* March 2, 2016. https://www.1843magazine.com/features/why-do-we-work-so-hard.

Bhattarai, Abha. "Lego Sets Its Sights on a Growing Market: Stressed-Out Adults." *Washington Post,* January 16, 2020. https://www.washingtonpost.com/business/2020/01/16/legos-toys-for-stressed-adults.

Brody, Jane E. "The Health Benefits of Knitting." *New York Times,* January 25, 2016. https://well.blogs.nytimes.com/2016/01/25/the-health-benefits-of-knitting.

Chillag, Amy. "Why Adults Should Play, Too." CNN, November 2, 2017. https://edition.cnn.com/2017/11/02/health/why-adults-should-play-too/index.html.

Contie, Vicki. "Brain Imaging Reveals Joys of Giving." NIH Research Matters June 22, 2017. https://www.nih.gov/news-events/nih-research-matters/brain-imaging-reveals-joys-giving.

Csikszentmihalyi, Mihaly. *Flow: The Psychology of Optimal Experience.* HarperCollins Publishers, 1990.

Doepke, Matthias, and Fabrizio Zilibotti. *Love, Money, and Parenting: How Economics Explains the Way We Raise Our Kids.* Princeton University Press, 2019.

Fitzpatrick, Kelly. "Why Adult Coloring Books Are Good for You." CNN, August 1, 2017. https://edition.cnn.com/2016/01/06/health/adult-coloring-books-popularity-mental-health/index.html.

Gregoire, Carolyn. "Taking a Walk in Nature Could Be the Best Thing You Do for Your Mood All Day." *HuffPost,* September 23, 2014. https://www.huffpost.com/entry/walk-nature-depression_n_5870134.

Hauka, Lynn. "The Sweetness of Holding Space for Another." *HuffPost,* March 28, 2016. https://www.huffpost.com/entry/the-sweetness-of-holding-_b_9558266.

Kay, Jonathan. "The Invasion of the German Board Games." *The Atlan-*

tic, January 21, 2018. https://www.theatlantic.com/business /archive/2018/01/german-board-games-catan/550826.

"Keep Your Brain Young with Music." John Hopkins Medicine. https:// www.hopkinsmedicine.org/health/wellness-and-prevention/ keep-your-brain-young-with-music.

Marselle, Melissa R., Katherine N. Irvine, and Sara L. Warber. "Examining Group Walks in Nature and Multiple Aspects of Well-Being: A Large-Scale Study." *Ecopsychology,* September 19, 2014. https:// www.liebertpub.com/doi/full/10.1089/eco.2014.0027.

Newport, Cal. *Digital Minimalism: Choosing a Focused Life in a Noisy World.* Portfolio, 2019.

Plans, David. "We've Lost Touch with Our Bodies." *Scientific American,* February 5, 2019. https://blogs.scientificamerican.com/observations /weve-lost-touch-with-our-bodies.

Preidt, Robert. "Volunteering May Make People Happier, Study Finds." WebMD, August 23, 2013. https://www.webmd.com/balance /news/20130823/volunteering-may-make-people-happier-study -finds.

Santi, Jenny. "The Secret to Happiness Is Helping Others." *Time,* August 4, 2017. https://time.com/collection/guide-to-happiness /4070299/secret-to-happiness.

"Stress Management: Relaxing Your Mind and Body." *Healthwise.* https://www.uofmhealth.org/health-library/uz2209.

"Why Sitting May Be Hazardous to Your Health." *Harvard Women's Health Watch,* October 17, 2016. https://www.health.harvard.edu /staying-healthy/why-sitting-may-be-hazardous-to-your-health.

EPILOGUE: Creating Nikstopia

Bregman, Rutger. *Utopia for Realists: How We Can Build the Ideal World.* Little, Brown, 2017.

Carrington, Damian. "Climate Emergency: World 'May Have Crossed Tipping Points.'" *Guardian,* November 27, 2019. https://www

.theguardian.com/environment/2019/nov/27/climate-emergency
-world-may-have-crossed-tipping-points.

Cellan-Jones, Rory. "Robots 'To Replace Up to 20 Million Factory
Jobs' by 2030." BBC, June 26, 2019. https://www.bbc.com/news
/business-48760799.

Coontz, Stephanie. *The Way We Never Were: American Families and
the Nostalgia Trap.* Basic Books, 1992.

Crabbe, Tony. *Busy: How to Thrive in a World of Too Much.* Piatkus,
2014.

Dell'Antonia, K. J. "I Refuse to Be Busy." *New York Times,* April 3, 2014.
https://parenting.blogs.nytimes.com/2014/04/03/i-refuse-to-be
-busy.

Dockray, Heather. "Self-Care Isn't Enough. We Need Community Care
to Thrive." *Mashable,* May 24, 2019. https://mashable.com/article
/community-care-versus-self-care.

Fishman, Noam, and Alyssa Davis. "Americans Still See Big Government as Top Threat." Gallup, January 5, 2017. https://news.gallup
.com/poll/201629/americans-big-government-top-threat.aspx.

Glass, Jennifer. "Parenting and Happiness in 22 Countries." Council of
Contemporary Families, June 16, 2016. https://contemporary
families.org/brief-parenting-happiness.

Hopkins, Rob. *From What Is to What If: Unleashing the Power of Imagination to Create the Future We Want.* Chelsea Green Publishing,
2019.

Khazan, Olga. "Why Some Cultures Frown on Smiling." *The Atlantic,*
May 27, 2016. https://www.theatlantic.com/science/archive/2016
/05/culture-and-smiling/483827.

Kuipers Munneke, Peter. "De vraag is niet óf Nederland onder water
verdwijnt, maar waneer." *NRC,* July 13, 2018. https://www.nrc.nl
/next/2018/07/13/#120.

Mecking, Olga. "Are the Floating Houses of the Netherlands a Solution
Against the Rising Seas?" *Pacific Standard,* August 21, 2017.
https://psmag.com/environment/are-the-floating-houses-of
-the-netherlands-a-solution-against-the-rising-seas.

———. "The Polish Phrase That Will Help You Through Tough Times." BBC, November 8, 2017. http://www.bbc.com/travel/story/20171107 -the-polish-phrase-that-will-help-you-through-tough-times.

Pew Research Center. "Majorities Say Government Does Too Little for Older People, the Poor and the Middle Class." January 30, 2018. https://www.people-press.org/2018/01/30/majorities-say -government-does-too-little-for-older-people-the-poor-and -the-middle-class.

Rankin, Jennifer. "'Our House Is on Fire': EU Parliament Declares Climate Emergency." *Guardian,* November 28, 2019. https://www .theguardian.com/world/2019/nov/28/eu-parliament-declares -climate-emergency.

Ratcliffe, Glynis. "Eco-Anxiety Isn't New, and It's Time to Deal with It." *Asparagus,* February 5, 2019. https://medium.com/asparagus -magazine/eco-anxiety-climate-change-coping-treatment-cbt -72625b481f54.

Smedley, Tim. "How Shorter Workweeks Could Save Earth." BBC, August 7, 2019. https://www.bbc.com/worklife/article/20190802 -how-shorter-workweeks-could-save-earth.

Wolff, Jonathan. "Technology Just Makes Us All Busier." *Guardian,* November 7, 2011. https://www.theguardian.com/education/2011 /nov/07/time-saving-technology.

Younge, Gary. "In These Bleak Times, Imagine a World Where You Can Thrive." *Guardian,* January 10, 2020. https://www.theguardian .com/commentisfree/2020/jan/10/bleak-times-thrive-last-column -guardian.

Index

Index

(249)

Index